HUMAN OSTEOLOGY

(TEXT AND COLOUR ATLAS)

HUMAN OSTEOLOGY
(TEXT AND COLOUR ATLAS)

GP PAL

MBBS, MS, DSc, FAMS, FNASc, FASc

Prof and Head

Dept of Anatomy

Modern Dental College and Research Center

Indore, Madhya Pradesh, India

Formerly

Professor and Head

Dept of Anatomy

MP Shah Medical College

Jamnagar, Gujarat

Formerly

Visiting Associate Professor

Dept of Anatomy

The Medical College of Pennsylvania

Philadelphia, USA

PEEPEE
PUBLISHERS AND DISTRIBUTORS (P) LTD.

Human Osteology
(Text and Colour Atlas)

Published by
Pawaninder P. Vij

Peepee Publishers and Distributors (P) Ltd.
Head Office: 160, Shakti Vihar, Pitam Pura, Delhi-110 034 (India)
Corporate Office: **7/31, First Floor, Ansari Road, Daryaganj**
Post Box-7243, New Delhi-110002 (India)
Ph: 65195868, 23246245, 9811156083
e-mail: peepee160@yahoo.co.in
e-mail: peepee160@rediffmail.com
e-mail: peepee160@gmail.com
www.peepeepub.com

This book has been published in good faith that the material provided by authors/contributors is original. Every effort is made to ensure accuracy of material, but publisher and printer will not be held responsible for any inadvertent errors. In case of any dispute, all legal matters to be settled under Delhi jurisdiction only.

First Edition: **2011**

ISBN: 81-8445-091-5

Printed at: Lordson, C-5/19, Rana Pratap Bagh, Delhi-110 007

Dedicated
to
Vedant and Yathaarth

Preface

Osteology is an important branch of gross anatomy. Without a sound knowledge of bones it is impossible to understand the gross anatomy of the body. Osteology was taught in great details in India till recent past. However, due to reduction in the duration of undergraduate studies, now it is difficult to cope up with the detail study of each and every bone. The unnecessary details of the bones also become irrelevant due to increasing use of CT scan and MRI. This book has been produced to fulfill the present day need of our students.

- The book is profusely illustrated. The legends and labeling of diagrams are such that they help in understanding the text easily.
- As it is becoming increasingly difficult to procure the human bones, labeled photographs of high resolution are given in the book. This will help students to understand areas of bone, which are difficult to visualize and appreciate through diagrams.
- To make the subject interesting, relevant clinical conditions are presented in simple language under the heading "Clinical Importance".
- Minimum text is given to describe the attachment of muscles, ligaments and articular capsules. Students can learn this with the help of well-labeled diagrams. Similarly, ossification of bone is depicted through diagrams.
- New information is presented under separate heading "Further Details". This will be of help to postgraduate students.
- Similarly, findings from the research of author are also incorporated in "Further Details" that will provide clues to postgraduate students and research workers for further research on the subject.

Though all efforts have been made to minimize the errors, still many must have remained in the text. I would highly appreciate and welcome the suggestions for improvement.

Indore
October, 2010

GP Pal

Acknowledgements

I took the help of many people in the preparation of this book. I sincerely thank them all. I gratefully acknowledge the help and cooperation received from Dr R Badlani (Chairman, Modern Dental College and RC, Indore) and Dean, Dr PV Wanjari. My thanks are due to my colleagues in the department Dr (Mrs) S Choudhary and Dr (Mrs) Sonali Agichani for help in proof reading.

For drawing the large number of diagrams, I was assisted by many professional artists and my past students. I sincerely thank them all. These are: Miss Sneha Gupta, Miss Vishakha Rahatekar, Mrs Rajni Panwar, Miss Niti Pandit, Miss Hemali Patel, Miss Amrita Soni and Miss Sonam Agrawal. I also thank Mrs R Gupta, librarian, MDC and RC, for help extended in library related assistance.

I am highly thankful to my devoted wife Pushpa and other family members (Sandeep and Vedant) for their patience, love, understanding and support.

It has been my pleasure to work with Mr Pawaninder P Vij, Director and the staff of Peepee Publishers and Distributors (P) Ltd. who were all very friendly and cooperative throughout the preparation of this manuscript.

Indore
October, 2010

GP Pal

Contents

1 Introduction

The subject of "Human Anatomy" is mainly studied with the help of dissection of cadavers (dead bodies). The structure of various parts of body (i.e., muscles, blood vessels, nerves, joints and organs) and their interrelationship can be easily seen by the dissection of dead bodies. All these soft structures are arranged around in relation to bones, i.e., muscles and ligaments are attached to bones while, nerves, vessels and other soft structures are related (or present) close to the bones. It should also be realized that bones form skeletal framework of the body, therefore, give shape to the body. Hence, for proper understanding of the gross anatomy of any region it is essential to learn the structure of bones of that region first, i.e., before starting the dissection of that region. *Students should note that gross anatomy can't be learnt without the sound knowledge of osteology.*

What is Osteology?

Osteology is a branch of gross anatomy, which deals with the study of bones.

PARTS OF THE SKELETAL SYSTEM

The skeletal system consists of bones and cartilages. The cartilage is present at the ends of bone. The skeletal system consists of two main parts, i.e., axial and appendicular skeleton.

The Axial Skeleton

It consists of bones lying close to the central axis of the body, e.g., skull, vertebrae, sacrum, coccyx, hyoid bone, sternum and ribs.

The Appendicular Skeleton

It consists of the bones of the upper limb and lower limb including bones forming shoulder and pelvic girdles.

How many bones are present in a human skeleton?

There are approximately about 206 bones present in an adult human. Out of these 80 are present in axial skeleton and 126 in the appendicular skeleton (Table 1.1).

Table 1.1: Number of bones present in axial and appendicular skeleton			
Axial skeleton		Appendicular skeleton	
Skull bones	22	Shoulder girdles	4
Vertebrae	26	(Right and left)	
Sternum	1	Pelvic girdles	2
Hyoid	1	Upper limb	60
Ribs	24	Lower limb	60
Auditory ossicles	6		
(3 on each side)			
Total	80	Total	126

The total number of bones in human body may exceed 206. This is due to the fact that some accessory (supernumerary) bones may appear especially in skull and lower limbs.

BONE STRUCTURE

Bone is a dynamic living tissue of the body. It is a constantly changing tissue, i.e., old bone tissues are constantly replaced by new ones. Bone is composed of cells and intercellular matrix. Bundles of collagen fibers are embedded in the matrix. It is hard because of deposition of calcium salts in the matrix.

Gross (Macroscopic) Structure of An Adult Living Long Bone

A typical long bone (bone of limb) consists of a *shaft* or *body* and two *ends* (Fig. 1.1). Both the ends of a bone are knobby (enlarged) and are covered by articular cartilage. The shaft of a long bone lies between two ends. It is narrow in middle and expanded towards each end. It encloses a cavity called as *marrow cavity*, which in an adult is filled with yellow bone marrow. The entire bone is covered with a fibrous membrane (*periosteum*) except at the areas covered by *articular cartilage*. Blood vessels and nerves enter the bone through numerous foramina present near the ends and at middle of the shaft. The prominent foramen of the shaft is called as nutrient foramen.

Further details of a living long bone may be studied by observing a longitudinal section of any long bone from upper or lower limb. The section reveals two different kinds of bones, i.e., *compact* and *spongy* (Fig. 1.2).

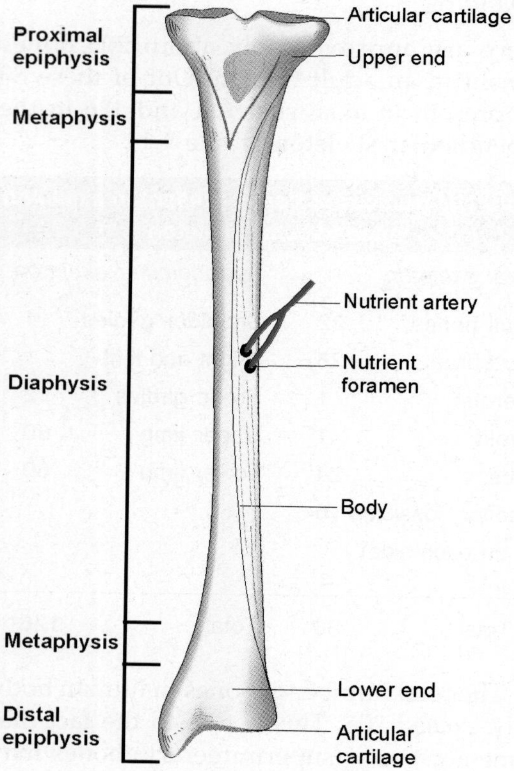

Compact Bone

The compact bone is a dense bone in which no spaces are visible on naked eye examination. Its texture is like an ivory. Though the compact bone covers the entire bone it is well developed in the shaft or body. The compact bone of the shaft encloses the marrow cavity filled with bone marrow.

Fig. 1.1: The parts of a long bone

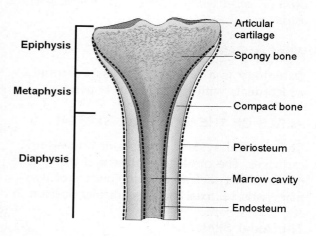

Fig. 1.2: Longitudinal section of a long bone to show compact and spongy bones and various other parts

Spongy or Trabecular Bone

It is also known as cancellous bone. Spongy bone is a meshwork of bony spicules (small rods and thin curved plates), which encloses large spaces. The spongy bone occurs at the ends of a long bone. On the outer surface, the spongy bone is always covered with a thin layer of compact bone. The spaces between spicules are filled with red bone marrow.

FURTHER DETAILS

Spongy Bone

The details about spongy bone is out of the scope of this book. Postgraduate students are advised to refer to the following three publications for structure and function of spongy bone:
- I. Singh (1978) *J. of Anatomy* (U.K.) 127: 305-310.
- G.P. Pal (1988) *The Anatomical Record* (New York) 222: 418-425.
- G.P. Pal (1990) *The J. of ASI* 39: 1-11.

Parts of a Living Long Bone

From the above description it becomes evident that a living long bone consists of following parts:
- Shaft or body (Diaphysis and Metaphyses).
- Two ends (Epiphyses).
- Articular cartilage.
- Periosteum.
- Endosteum.
- Medullary cavity.
- Bone marrow.

1. Shaft or Body

The shaft of a long bone is a long, cylindrical (tubular) structure, made up of compact bone. It is also called as *diaphysis*. It encloses a tubular space called as marrow cavity. The compact bone of shaft provides support and bears the weight. It is also capable of resisting the various stress produced by movements.

The expanded distal ends of shaft or body, where they meet with the articular ends *(epiphyses)*, are called as *metaphyses*.

2. Two Ends

Two ends (proximal and distal) are expanded and made up of spongy bone covered with a thin layer of compact bone. At ends, a long bone forms synovial joints and thus come in contact with other bones. The ends are covered by hyaline cartilage. This articular end of a long bone is also called as *epiphysis*.

3. Articular Cartilage

As stated earlier the ends of a long bone are covered by a thin layer of hyaline cartilage at the site where bone comes in contact with other bone (forms a joint). The articular cartilage provides smooth surface thus reduces friction between two bones during movements. It also helps in absorption of shock during movements.

4. Periosteum

The entire outer surface of bone (except where it is covered by articular cartilage) is covered with a tough sheath of dense connective tissue. This membrane is attached to the bone tissue by *Sharpey's fibers*. The periosteum consists of an outer layer of collagen fibers and fibroblasts and an inner layer of fibroblasts like cells called as osteoprogenitor cells. The osteoprogenitor cells have the potential to divide and change to osteoblasts (bone forming cells). The periosteum serves the following functions:
- It forms an outer limit of bone, thus maintains its shape. It also protects the bone.
- Periosteum contains bone-forming cells, which helps bone to grow in diameter.

- It is richly supplied with blood vessels thus helps in providing nutrition to bone and assists in fracture repair.
- It is also richly supplied with sensory nerves, making it sensitive to pain.
- Periosteum provides attachment to ligaments, tendons, muscles, intermuscular septa and articular capsule of a joint.

5. Endosteum

Endosteum is a cellular membrane that lines the medullary cavity of shaft and the medullary spaces of spongy bone at ends. It is composed of a single layer of flattened osteoprogenitor cells and very small amount of connective tissue.

6. Medullary or Marrow Cavity

It is a space within the shaft or body of a long bone. The marrow cavity of shaft is continuous with the spaces of spongy bone at ends.

7. Bone Marrow

The marrow cavity of a newborn is filled with red bone marrow that is actively involved in the formation of blood. Red bone marrow consists of adipose and haemopoietic (blood forming) tissues. However, with the advancing age the red marrow in the shaft of bone is replaced by yellow marrow (fatty marrow), which is unable to produce blood cells. In adults, red marrow only remains at the ends of long bones, sternum ribs, skull bones and vertebrae. At these places red marrow is actively involved in production of blood cells throughout the life.

SOME IMPORTANT FACTS ABOUT THE BONE

Students should note that the above description is of a living bone (bone present in a living person). They should realize that the bones, which they handle in classroom, are dry and devoid of many structural components of a living bone. For example, a dry bone is not covered by hyaline cartilage at its epiphyseal ends. Similarly, it is also devoid of periosteum, endosteum, bone marrow, blood vessels and nerves. Bone is not only a living tissue but it is also a dynamic tissue. It is continuously engaged in building new bone and breaking down the old bone.

Students should also realize that each individual living bone is not just a bone tissue but somewhat similar to an organ. It is evident by the fact that a bone consists of not only bone tissue proper but also consists many other tissues like fibrous membranes (periosteum and endosteum), cartilage (articular cartilage), bone marrow (adipose and haemopoietic tissues), nerves and blood vessels. Similar to any other organ of body, bone is also involved in various functional activities (locomotion, support and protection of delicate organs, formation of blood and storage of calcium).

FEATURES ON THE SURFACE OF DRY BONE (BONE MARKINGS)

In your osteology classroom, you will handle the dead dried bones to learn their general features. The structures, which are attached to a bone or are in close contact with it, in living condition, leave the marks on the bone surface. Following kinds of bony features (smooth areas, surface elevations, surface depressions and foramina) can be observed on the surface of dried bones:

A. Smooth Areas

The smooth areas on a bone are found at places where it gives attachment to muscle fibers; where it is covered by articular cartilage; and where it lies directly beneath the skin in living condition.

Facet

It is a flat and smooth area on the bone (Fig. 1.3). In living state it is covered with articular cartilage, e.g., articular facets on the surface of carpal and tarsal bones.

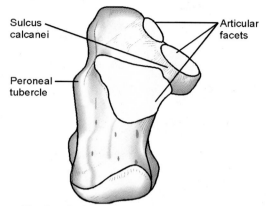

Fig. 1.3: Articular facets on the calcaneus

B. Surface Elevations

These are of many types, i.e., crest, line, lip and ridge are elongated surface elevations. While tubercle, tuberosity, epicondyle and trochanter are irregular elevations. These surface elevations are mostly due to the attachment of tendons, ligaments or aponeurosis. Some surface elevations are sharp like spine, cornu or styloid process.

Features	Description
Crest:	It is a bony ridge, which may be quite wide, e.g., the iliac crest of hip bone (Fig. 1.4) or narrow, e.g., external occipital crest (Fig. 1.7).

Fig. 1.4: The iliac crest of hip bone

Line: An elevated line on the surface of bone, e.g., the soleal line of tibia (Fig. 1.5) and superior nuchal line of occipital bone (Fig. 1.7).

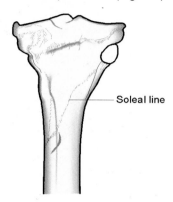

Fig. 1.5: The soleal line of tibia

Condyle: A bony mass, which may have somewhat rounded or circular articular area, e.g., condyles of femur (Fig. 1.6).

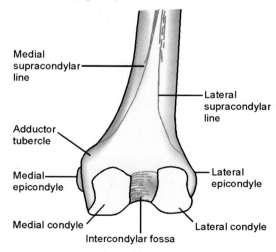

Fig. 1.6: Condyles, epicondyles and tubercle at the lower end of femur

Epicondyle: Bony eminence (protuberance) situated on the surface of the condyle, e.g., lateral and medial epicondyle of femur (Fig. 1.6).

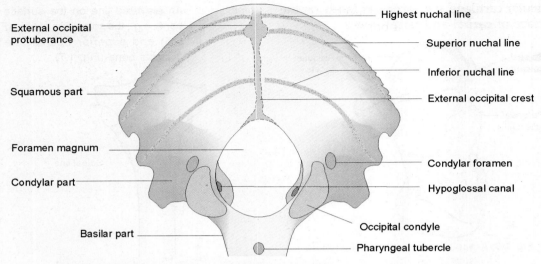

Fig. 1.7: The occipital bone showing crest, nuchal lines and protuberance

Protub-erance:	A projection from the surface of the bone, e.g., the external occipital protuberance (Fig. 1.7).
Malleolus:	It is a rounded bony process, e.g., the medial malleolus of fibia (Fig. 1.8).
Spinous process:	A spine like projection, e.g., the spinous process of a vertebra (Fig. 1.9).
Trochanter:	It is a large blunt elevation from the surface of bone, e.g., greater and lesser trochanters of femur (Fig. 1.10).

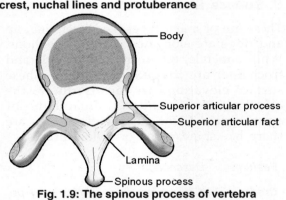

Fig. 1.9: The spinous process of vertebra

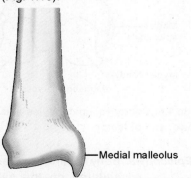

Fig. 1.8: Large, rounded elevation of tibia, i.e., malleolus

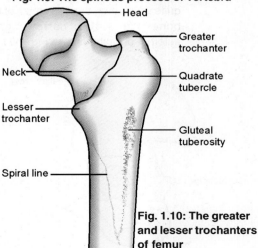

Fig. 1.10: The greater and lesser trochanters of femur

Tuberosity: A large rounded elevation, e.g., the ischial tuberosity (Figs. 1.11 and 1.12).

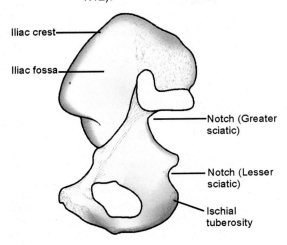

Iliac crest

Iliac fossa

Notch (Greater sciatic)

Notch (Lesser sciatic)

Ischial tuberosity

Fig. 1.11: Tuberosity is a large elevation while notch is a deep indentation

Tubercle: A raised elevation, but smaller than trochanter, e.g., adductor tubercle of femur (Fig. 1.6).

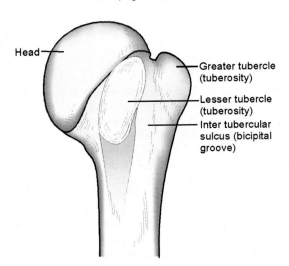

Head

Greater tubercle (tuberosity)

Lesser tubercle (tuberosity)

Inter tubercular sulcus (bicipital groove)

Fig. 1.12: The bicipital groove of humerus is the elongated depression

C. Surface Depressions and Foramina

Groove or sulcus: It is an elongated depression on the surface of bone, e.g., bicipital groove of humerus (Fig. 1.12).

The groove or sulcus on a dry bone indicates that the bone in living condition was in relation to blood vessels or tendon.

Notch: It is a deep indentation at the border of a bone, e.g., greater and lesser sciatic notches of hip bone (Fig. 1.11) and suprascapular notch of scapula (Fig. 1.13).

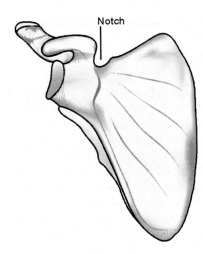

Notch

Fig. 1.13: Notch at the upper border of scapula

Fossa: A depression on the surface of bone, e.g., illiac fossa of hip bone and olecranon fossa of humerus (Figs. 1.11 and 1.14).

Foramina: Bones show many openings on the surface, i.e., canals and foramina.

A canal is a tunnel like passage with one opening at each end. These are usually for passage of blood vessels and nerves.

A bone may also show some other surface features, which you must learn with the help of your teachers.

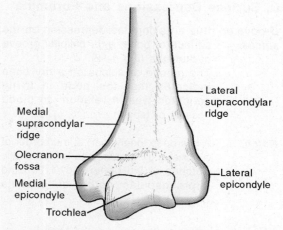

Medial supracondylar ridge

Lateral supracondylar ridge

Olecranon fossa

Lateral epicondyle

Medial epicondyle

Trochlea

Fig. 1.14: The olecranon fossa at the lower end of humerus

HOW TO STUDY A BONE?

Following guidelines will be of help when you are learning any particular bone for the first time.

- While you are studying a bone you should have the same bone before you. There is no sense in reading about a bone, from a book, without having that bone in your hand.
- First step in learning a bone is to identify its ends (upper end, lower end etc.), borders and surfaces. This can be learned with the help of your teachers or with the help of diagrams from this book.
- Second step is to identify some of the important projections (e.g., spine, tubercle, ridge, condyle etc.) and depressions (e.g., fossa, foramen, notch etc.), if present on the bone.

Side Determination of the Bone

- Once you have identified the ends, borders and surfaces and some of bony features you would be able to determine the side of bone. Take the help of your teachers to know which are the bony features of that particular bone which will help to determine

the side of bone. (In case of bones belonging to axial skeleton there is no need to determine the side as many of them are unpaired, i.e., some bones of skull, vertebrae etc.). *Side determination of the bone is very important.*

Anatomical Position

- Next step is to learn to hold the bone in anatomical position. Once you have determined the side of the bone hold it in the position as it occupies in the body (as in anatomical position). All the description of the bone in the textbooks is given considering the position of bone in upright posture (anatomical position). If the bone, while studying, is not held in anatomical position, confusion will arise regarding its borders and surfaces.

General Features

- Now learn the bony features ("General Features") of bone in detail. After understanding the general feature it will become very easy to know the side of the bone and to keep it in the anatomical position.

Particular Features

- Once you have understood the general features of a bone it is now time to study the "particular features" (attachments of muscles and ligaments and relations of nerves and vessels). This can be practised by marking the area of origin of muscle by a red chalk and insertion of muscle by a blue chalk on the surface of bone. All the sites for attachments of ligaments should be marked with green chalk. Mark the area of bone, which is in relation to nerve, by a solid line with yellow chalk. Similarly, the relation of artery and vein on the surface of a bone can be marked with the red and blue lines respectively.

Ossification

- You may also study the ossification of bone, *if needed. (Ask your teacher whether you are supposed to know the ossification or not?).* Note the age of appearance of primary center, secondary centers and time of fusion of primary with secondary centers. Also note which end of a long bone is a *"**growing end**"*. Students are suggested to learn about the **"ossification"** and **"growing end of bone"** from a book of "General Anatomy".

Clinical Importance

- Lastly you should also learn **"applied"** or **"clinical importance"** of the bone, if any.

2 Bones of the Upper Limb

The upper limb consists of many regions. Following bones are present in various regions of the upper limb (Fig. 2.1):

Pectoral Region

It consists of two bones on each side, i.e., *clavicle* and *scapula*. These two bones form the pectoral or shoulder girdle. The lateral end of clavicle articulates with the scapula at *acromio-clavicular joint*. The medial end of clavicle articulates with sternum (axial skeleton) through *sterno-clavicular joint*. Thus the pectoral girdle serves to attach the upper limb to trunk.

Arm

This region consists of single bone called as *humerus*. The upper end of this bone articulates with scapula at shoulder joint. The lower end of humerus articulates with two long bones of forearm, i.e., radius and ulna at elbow joint.

Forearm

The *ulna* is medial while *radius* is laterally placed in forearm. At their lower ends they articulate with carpal bones to form wrist joint.

Hand

The skeleton of hand consists of many bones, i.e., *carpals*, *metacarpals* and *phalanges*. These

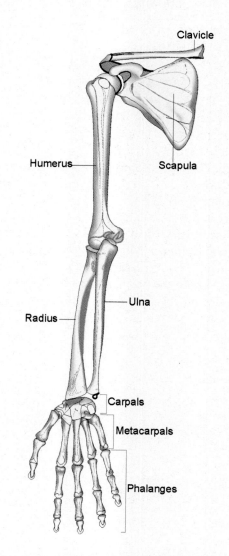

Fig. 2.1: Schematic diagram to show the bones of the right upper limb

bones form many joints i.e., intercarpal, carpometacarpal, metacarpophalangeal and interphalangeal joints.

THE CLAVICLE

The description of the bone in the following paragraph and the reference to Figs. 2.2 and 2.3 will help you to learn the "side determination" and "anatomical position" of bone.

The clavicle (collar bone) is an horizontally placed long bone, which shows two ends (medial and lateral) and a shaft (Figs. 2.2 and 2.3). The medial end is thick and rounded while lateral end is broad and flattened. The shaft shows "S" shaped double curvatures, which meet each other at the junction of medial 2/3 and lateral 1/3 of the bone. The medial 2/3 of the bone is cylindrical and convex forwards, while lateral 1/3 of the shaft is flattened and concave forwards. The superior surface of the bone is smooth as it is subcutaneous. On the other hand, inferior surface is rough near its medial and lateral ends due to the attachment of ligaments. The inferior surface also shows the presence of a shallow groove in its middle third.

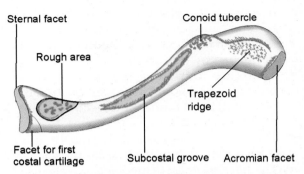

Fig. 2.3: General features of inferior surface of right clavicle

Side Determination

- Hold the bone horizontally in such a way that its rounded thick end is nearer to the median plane (placed medially) and flattened end is directed laterally.
- Identify the rough inferior surface and smooth superior surface. Keep the inferior surface facing inferiorly (towards ground).
- The convexity of medial 2/3 of shaft should be directed anteriorly.
- In this position the lateral end will direct the side of bone.

Anatomical Position

Hold the clavicle horizontally in such a way that its medial end is directed slightly forward and inferiorly as compared to its lateral end (which is directed upward and backward).

General Features

For the ease of understanding the clavicle is divided into medial 2/3 and lateral 1/3.

Medial 2/3 of Clavicle

Hold the bone in anatomical position and note the following (Fig. 2.2):

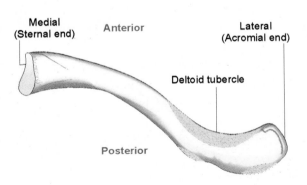

Fig. 2.2: General features of superior surface of right clavicle

- It consists of cylindrical shaft and thick rounded medial (sternal) end.
- As the shaft is cylindrical borders are ill defined (not well marked).
- There are four surfaces, i.e., superior, inferior, anterior and posterior. In absence of well-defined borders these surfaces are continuous with each other.
- The *superior surface* is mostly smooth. It is covered by skin and *platysma* muscle.
- The *anterior surface* of medial 2/3 of clavicle is convex anteriorly.
- The *posterior surface* is smooth and concave posteriorly.

Now turn the bone upside down so as to see the inferior surface (Fig. 2.3).

- The *inferior surface* has a large rough impression near its medial end, which gives attachment to a ligament.
- There is presence of a shallow groove in the middle third of the inferior surface. This groove is known as *subclavian groove*.

The medial end of clavicle shows a large smooth saddle shaped articular surface on its medial aspect (*sternal surface*), which also extends for a short distance on the inferior surface of the bone. The medial end of the clavicle articulates with the manubrium sterni (at *sternoclavicular joint*) and also with the first costal cartilage near its inferior surface.

Lateral 1/3 of the Clavicle

As the lateral 1/3 of the clavicle is flat. It shows well-defined anterior and posterior borders and superior and inferior surfaces.

Hold the bone in the anatomical position and note the following (Fig. 2.2):
- The *anterior border* is concave forwards and shows a small rough area called as *deltoid tubercle*.
- The *posterior border* is rough and convex posteriorly.
- The superior surface is mostly smooth except near its anterior and posterior

borders, which give attachment to muscles.

Now turn the bone upside down so as to see the inferior surface of lateral 1/3 (Fig. 2.3).

- The inferior surface near its posterior border shows a tubercle known as *conoid tubercle.*
- A thick ridge extends forward and laterally from the conoid tubercle. This ridge is known as *trapezoid ridge.*

The lateral end of the bone bears a small oval facet for articulation with the acromian process of the scapula to form *acromio-clavicular joint.*

Particular Features

Muscles Attached to Bone

Draw the attachments of muscles on the surface of bone with the help of colored chalk as shown in Figures 2.4 and 2.5.

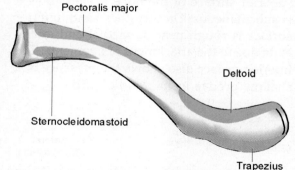

Fig. 2.4: Attachment of muscles on superior surface

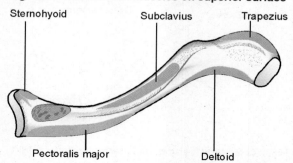

Fig. 2.5: Attachment of muscles on inferior surface

Medial 2/3 of Clavicle

- The superior surface is covered by skin and *platysma* muscle. The clavicular head of *sternocleidomastoid* muscle arises from the medial third of this surface (Fig. 2.4).
- The anterior surface of medial half of clavicle gives origin to the clavicular head of *pectoralis major.*
- The muscle *sternohyoid* is attached near the medial end of the posterior surface of the clavicle.
- On the inferior surface, the *subclavius* muscle is attached in the subclavian groove (Fig. 2.5).
- The margins of this groove give attachment to *clavipectoral fascia* (Fig. 2.7A).

Lateral 1/3 of the Clavicle

- The anterior border gives origin to the *deltoid muscle.*
- Posterior border gives attachment to the *trapezius muscle.*

Ligaments Attached to Bone

- The attachments of *articular capsule* at its medial and lateral ends are shown in Figs. 2.6 and 2.7.
- The *costoclavicular ligament* is attached on the inferior rough surface near its medial end (Fig. 2.7B).

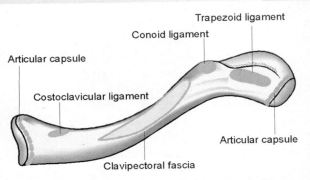

Fig. 2.7A: Inferior surface showing attachment of ligaments

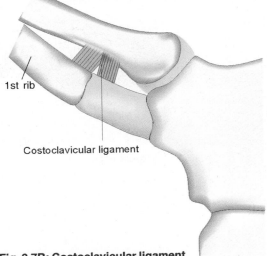

Fig. 2.7B: Costoclavicular ligament

- *Interclavicular ligament* and the articular disc of sternoclavicular joint are attached on medial surface of the medial end.
- Conoid and trapezoid parts of the *coracoclavicular ligament* are attached on the conoid tubercle and trapezoid ridge respectively on the inferior surface of lateral 1/3.

Nerves and Blood Vessels Related to Bone

- Three *supra-clavicular nerves* (medial, intermediate and lateral) are related to its anterosuperior surface (Fig. 2.6).

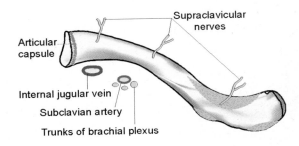

Fig. 2.6: Superior surface of clavicle showing attachment of ligaments and relation of nerves

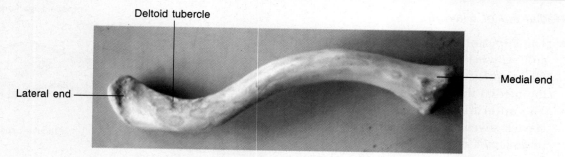

Deltoid tubercle

Lateral end

Medial end

Fig. 2A: Superior view of left clavicle

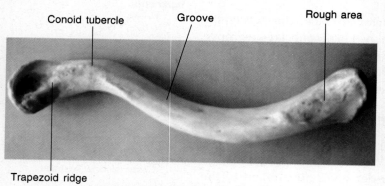

Conoid tubercle

Groove

Rough area

Trapezoid ridge

Fig. 2B: Inferior view of left clavicle

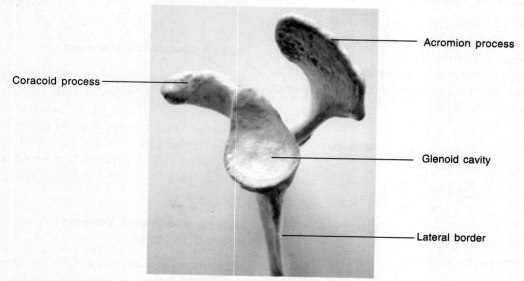

Acromion process

Coracoid process

Glenoid cavity

Lateral border

Fig. 2C: Lateral aspect of the left scapula

- The posterior surface of medial 2/3 of shaft is related to the trunks of brachial plexus, third part of *subclavian vessels* and *internal jugular vein.*

Peculiarities of the Clavicle

- Though it is a long bone but is placed horizontally.
- Though long bone but ossifies mostly from membrane.
- It is devoid of medullary cavity.
- First bone to start ossifying in the body.

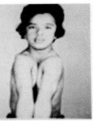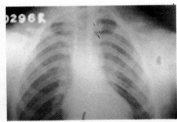

- The concave posterior surface of medial 2/3 of the bone protects the nerves and vessels (trunks of brachial plexus and subclavian vessels), which go from the root of the neck to the axilla (Fig. 2.6).

CLINICAL APPLICATION

- The main function of the clavicle is to transmit the forces from the upper limb to the axial skeleton through sternoclavicular joint. The forces are transmitted from humerus to scapula and then from scapula to clavicle through coracoclavicular ligament. If the force, during a fall on the outstretched hand, is greater than the strength of clavicle, a fracture will result at the junction between two curvatures of bone (medial 2/3 and lateral 1/3). After the fracture the shoulder drops and lateral fragment of clavicle is displaced downward due to the weight of upper limb (gravity). The medial fragment of bone is pulled upward due to the action of clavicular head of sternocleidomastoid muscle. The lateral fragment of the bone may also be pulled medially by the action of pectoralis major. Thus two fragments may override each other (Fig. 2.8). To approximate the two fractured ends of the bone, a bandage in the shape of *figure of eight* is tied.
- The clavicle acts as a strut to keep the shoulder laterally. This helps the upper limb to swing clearly away from the trunk. In a congenital malformation known as *cleido-cranial dysostosis*, the clavicle is either absent or imperfectly developed. In this condition shoulder joint is not always placed laterally and can be brought in front of chest.

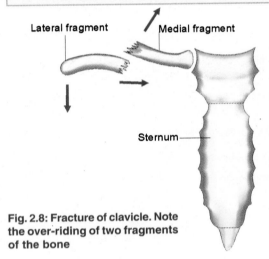

Fig. 2.8: Fracture of clavicle. Note the over-riding of two fragments of the bone

Ossification

The clavical is the first long lone to ossify in the embryo. It ossifies by two primary centers and one secondary center. Most of the shaft ossifies by membranous ossification (Fig. 2.9).

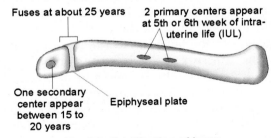

Fig. 2.9: Ossification of bone

THE SCAPULA

The description of the scapula in following two paragraphs and a reference to Figs. 2.10 and 2.11 will help you learn to determine its side and to keep it in the anatomical position.

The scapula is also known as "shoulder blade". It is the posterior bone of the shoulder girdle. It lies on the posterolateral aspect of thorax extending between 2nd and 7th rib. The body of the scapula is thin, flat and triangular in shape (Figs. 2.10 and 2.11).

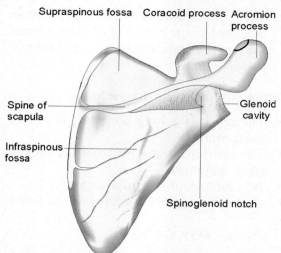

Fig. 2.11: Posterior (dorsal) surface of the right scapula

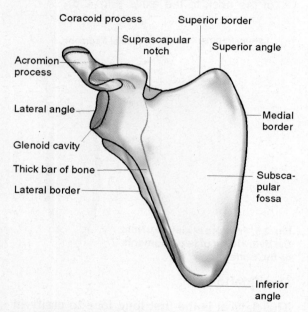

Fig. 2.10: Anterior (costal) surface of the right scapula

As the body is triangular in shape it has three borders (medial, lateral and superior) and three angles (superior, lateral and inferior). The inferior angle is directed downwards and lies at the level of 7th rib. Just opposite to the inferior angle is superior border, which extends between superior and lateral angles. At the lateral angle there is the presence of a shallow smooth articular fossa called as *glenoid cavity,* which articulates with the head of the humerus to form shoulder

joint. The medial border runs between superior and inferior angles and is quite thin. The lateral border is thick and runs between lateral and inferior angles.

The scapula shows two surfaces, i.e., costal and dorsal. The costal (anterior) surface is smooth and forms a shallow fossa called as *subscapular fossa*. On the other hand dorsal (posterior) surface is convex posteriorly and is divided into *supraspinous* and *infraspinous* fossae by the presence of a bony process called as *spine of the scapula.* It is a thick projecting ridge of bone, which is continuous laterally as the flat expanded *acromion process.* A beak like bony process (*coracoid process*) arises from the upper part of the glenoid cavity (Fig. 2.12).

Side Determination

Hold the bone in such a way that:
- The inferior angle is directed downwards and superior border is directed upwards.
- The costal or anterior surface should face anteriorly and the dorsal (posterior) surface, bearing the spinous process, should face posteriorly.
- The glenoid cavity should face laterally.

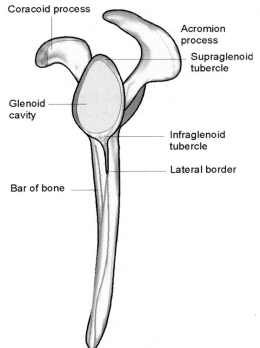

Coracoid process

Acromion process

Supraglenoid tubercle

Glenoid cavity

Infraglenoid tubercle

Lateral border

Bar of bone

Fig. 2.12: Lateral aspect of lelt scapula

- In this position the direction of glenoid cavity will determine the side of bone.

Anatomical Position

- Hold the bone in such a way that the costal surface should face antero-medially.
- The glenoid cavity should face antero-laterally and slightly upwards.

General Features

We shall study the general features of scapula under four different headings, i.e., surfaces, borders, angles and processes.

Surfaces

Costal (anterior) surface: The costal surface is slightly concave and forms a large *subscapular fossa.* There is presence of a bar of thickened bone near the lateral border extending between head of scapula (lateral angle) and inferior angle (Fig. 2.10).

Dorsal (posterior) surface: The spine of the scapula divides the dorsal surface into a smaller upper supraspinous fossa and a larger infraspinous fossa (Fig. 2.11). Both these fossae are continuous with each other through spinoglenoid notch.

Borders

Medial border: The medial border of the scapula is thin and lies about 5 cm lateral to the spinous processes of the thoracic vertebrae.

Lateral border: This border extends from the lowest part of the glenoid cavity to the inferior angle. It is a sharp ridge. Close to the lateral border, on the costal surface, there is presence of a thickened longitudinal bar of the bone (Fig. 2.10). It should not be confused with the lateral border.

Superior border: It extends between superior angle and the root of the coracoid process. This border presents a *suprascapular notch* close to the root of coracoid process.

Angles

The *superior* and *inferior angles* of the scapula are present at the upper and lower ends of the medial border respectively.

The lateral angle of the scapula is thickest part of the bone where glenoid cavity is present. This broadened part of the bone is sometimes called as *head* of the scapula. A constriction between head and body is called as *neck* of the scapula. The glenoid cavity is shallow, concave, oval fossa. There is presence of rough areas just above and below the glenoid cavity. These are called as *supraglenoid* and *infraglenoid* tubercles respectively (Fig. 2.12).

Processes

The *spine* of the scapula is a triangular bony process present on the dorsal aspect of the body. Its anterior border is attached to the dorsal surface of the body while its posterior border is free. This thick posterior border of the spine is also known as *crest of the spine*. The lateral border of spine forms the boundary of the spinoglenoid notch.

The *acromian process* is a forward projection from the lateral end of spine. It is a flat, expanded, subcutaneous process, which overhangs the glenoid cavity. It has medial and lateral borders and superior and inferior surfaces. It articulates with the lateral end of clavicle to form *acromioclavicular* joint.

The *coracoid process* is so named because it resembles to the beak of a crow. It is present superior to the glenoid cavity and is shaped like a bent finger (Fig. 2.10). In the anatomical position it projects anterolaterally.

Particular Features

Muscles Attached to Bone

Draw the attachments of muscles on the

surface of bone with the help of colored chalk as shown in Figures 2.13 and 2.14.

- Almost whole of the costal (anterior) surface (except a small part near the neck) gives origin to the *subscapularis* muscle.
- The medial border on the costal surface gives attachment to the *serratus anterior*.

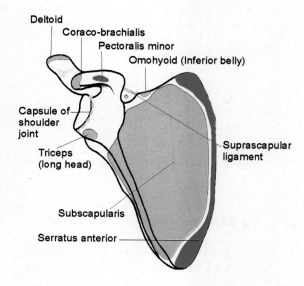

Fig. 2.13: Attachment of muscles on costal surface

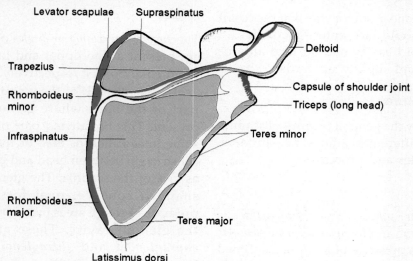

Fig. 2.14: Attachment of muscles on dorsal surface

- The *inferior belly of omohyoid* is attached on the superior border near the suprascapular notch.
- On the dorsal surface, the supraspinous fossa gives origin to *supraspinatus* muscle and infraspinous fossa to *infraspinatus* respectively (Fig. 2.14).
- The *teres major* and *teres minor* arise from the dorsal surface close to lateral border.
- Refer Fig. 2.14 to see the extent of attachments of *levator scapulae, rhomboideus minor* and *rhomboideus major* on the dorsal surface of the medial border.
- The supraglenoid tubercle gives origin to the long head of *biceps brachii*.
- *Long head of triceps* arises from the infraglenoid tubercle.
- *The coracobrachialis* and *short head of biceps* arises from the tip of coracoid process.
- *Pectoralis minor* is inserted on the superior aspect of coracoid process.
- The *deltoid muscle* arises from the lower border of the crest of spine and from the lateral border of acromion process.
- The medial border of the acromion and upper border of the crest of the spine gives insertion to the *trapezius*.

Ligaments Attached to Bone

- The attachments of the capsule of shoulder joint and acromioclavicular joints are shown in Figs. 2.13 and 2.14.
- The *suprascapular ligament* is attached on the superior border above the suprascapular notch (Fig. 2.15).
- Three ligaments are attached to the coracoid process, i.e., *coracohumeral, coracoacromial* and *coracoclavicular*. One end of the coracoacromial ligament is attached to lateral border of coracoid process and the other end to the tip of acromian process. The coracohumeral is attached to the root of coracoid process. The *conoid*

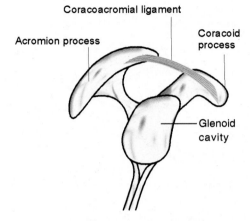

Fig. 2.15A: Attachments of ligaments

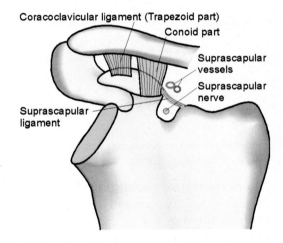

Fig. 2.15B: Attachments of ligaments

part of *coracoclavicular* ligament is attached near the root, while *trapezoid part* on the superior aspect of the coracoid process (Fig. 2.15).

Nerves and Blood Vessels Related to the Bone

- The *suprascapular vessels* lie above the suprascapular ligament, while *suprascapular nerve* passes deep to it (Fig. 2.15).
- These vessels and nerve then lie in spinoglenoid notch (Fig. 2.16).

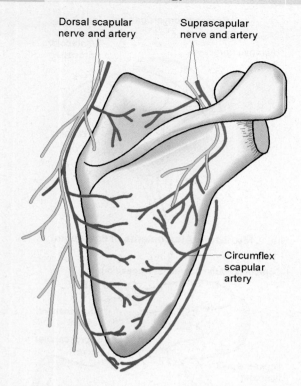

Fig. 2.16: Nerves and blood vessels related to scapula

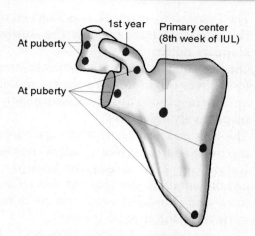

Fig. 2.17: Ossification of scapula

- The circumflex scapular branch of *subscapular artery* comes in contact with the lateral border on its dorsal aspect between two heads of teres minor (Fig. 2.16).
- The dorsal scapular nerve and vessels lie close to medial border.

Ossification

Scapula ossifies by one primary and 7 secondary centers (2 for coracoid process, 2 for acromion, 1 each for glenoid cavity, inferior angle and medial border) (Fig. 2.17). The lower center of coracoid process fuses with body by 16th year while other centers with the body by the end of 20th year.

HUMERUS

Humerus is the longest bone of the upper limb. It has two ends and a shaft (Figs. 2.18 and 2.19). The proximal (upper) end shows a large, smooth, rounded *head* that articulates with the glenoid cavity of the scapula to form the shoulder joint. The head is directed medially. There is presence of a deep vertical groove (*inter-tubercular sulcus* or *bicipital* groove) on the anterior aspect of the upper end. The middle part of shaft is almost cylindrical. The lower end is expanded from side to side and flattened from before backward. It has two articular structures, i.e., rounded *capitulum* and pulley shaped *trochlea*.

On the posterior aspect of lower end there is a large *olecranon fossa* just above the trochlea. The medial and lateral epicondyles are bony non-articular projections at the lower end.

Side Determination

- You should keep the bone vertical in such a way that the head faces medially.

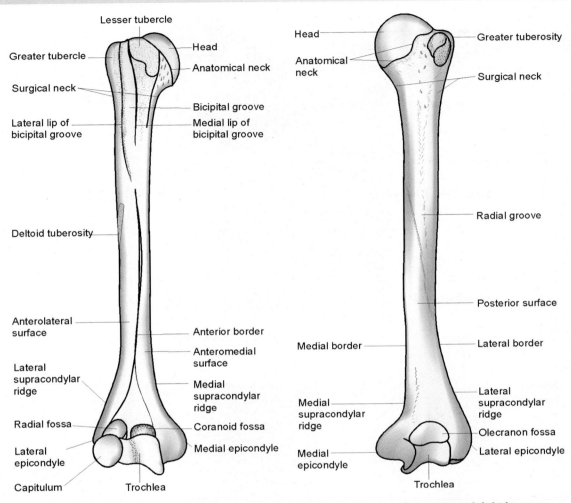

Fig. 2.18: Anterior aspect of right humerus

Fig. 2.19: Posterior aspect of right humerus

- The intertubercular sulcus on the anterior aspect of the upper end should face anteriorly.
- The olecranon fossa, at the lower end, should face posteriorly.

Anatomical Position

Hold the bone vertically in such a way that head faces medially and slightly upwards and backwards.

General Features

We shall study the general features of bone under three headings, i.e., upper end, shaft and lower end (Figs. 2.18 and 2.19).

Upper End

The upper end consists of head, neck, greater and lesser tubercles and an intertubercular sulcus (bicipital groove).

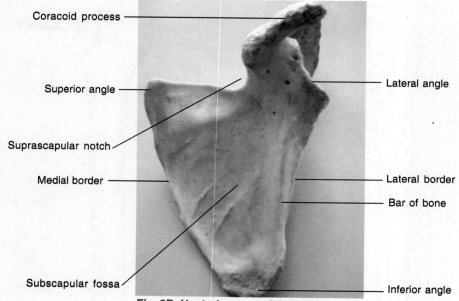

Coracoid process

Superior angle

Suprascapular notch

Medial border

Subscapular fossa

Lateral angle

Lateral border

Bar of bone

Inferior angle

Fig. 2D: Ventral aspect of the left scapula

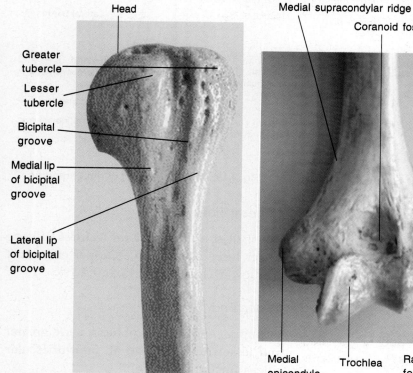

Head

Greater tubercle

Lesser tubercle

Bicipital groove

Medial lip of bicipital groove

Lateral lip of bicipital groove

Fig. 2E: Anterior aspect of upper end of left humerus

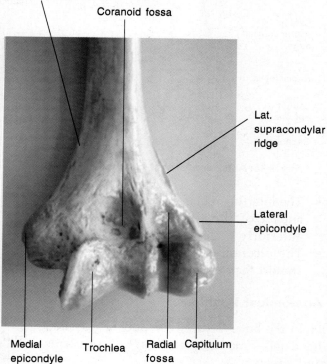

Medial supracondylar ridge

Coranoid fossa

Lat. supracondylar ridge

Lateral epicondyle

Medial epicondyle

Trochlea

Radial fossa

Capitulum

Fig. 2F: Anterior aspect of the lower end of left humerus

- The head has a convex, rounded and smooth articular surface.
- The junction of articular head with the rest of the upper end is called as *anatomical neck.*
- The junction of the upper expanded end with the shaft is called as *surgical neck.*
- The lesser tubercle is present on the anterior aspect of the upper end while greater tubercle is present on its anterolateral aspect.
- There is presence of intertubercular sulcus between these two tubercles.
- Both the tubercles on their upper surface show the presence of smooth areas for the attachment of muscles (Fig. 2.20).

Shaft

The shaft is almost cylindrical in upper half and triangular in lower half. It presents three borders and three surfaces.

Borders

- Trace the lateral lip of bicipital groove downward. You will see that it becomes continuous with the *anterior border* of the shaft (Fig. 2.18).
- The medial border of the bicipital groove is continuous downwards as the *medial border*. If this border is further traced downwards it becomes continuous as *medial supracondylar ridge.*

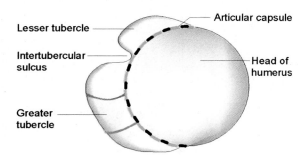

Fig. 2.20: Features on superior surface or upper end of right humerus

- The *lateral border* of the shaft is well defined only in lower part of the shaft where it becomes continuous with the *lateral supracondylar ridge.*

Surfaces

- The *anteromedial surface* is between anterior and medial border (Fig. 2.18).
- The *anterolateral* surface is between anterior and lateral borders. Just above the middle of bone this surface shows a V shaped rough area called as *deltoid tuberosity.*
- The *posterior surface* is situated between lateral and medial borders (Fig. 2.19). In its middle 1/3 it shows the presence of a shallow groove (*radial groove*) running downwards and laterally.

Lower End

- The lower end shows the presence of a rounded articular area known as capitulum. It is placed laterally and articulates with the upper end of radius.
- The pulley like trochlea is placed medially and articulates with the trochlear notch of ulna (Fig. 2.18).
- There is presence of shallow fossa above the capitulum (known as *radial fossa*) and *coronoid fossa* just above the trochlea. When forearm is flexed, the coronoid fossa and radial fossa receive coronoid process and head of radius respectively.
- The olecranon fossa is quite large and situated on the posterior surface of the lower end just above the trochlea. It receives the olecranon of ulna when forearm is extended (Fig. 2.19).
- If you will trace the medial and lateral supracondylar ridges downwards, you will reach the bony projections on either side of the lower end (Fig. 2.21). These rough projections are known as *epicondyles*. The medial epicondyle is the

prominent subcutaneous projection, which you should palpate (feel) in your own limb.

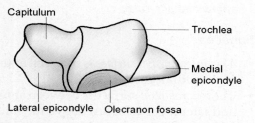

Fig. 2.21: The lower end of right humerus as seen from inferior aspect

Particular Features

Muscles Attached on Bone

Upper End

- The three impressions on the surface of greater tubercle give insertion *to supraspinatus, infraspinatus and teres minor* (Figs. 2.22 and 2.23).
- The *subscapularis* muscle is inserted on lesser tubercle (Fig. 2.22).
- The tendon of the long head of *biceps* passes through the bicipital groove.

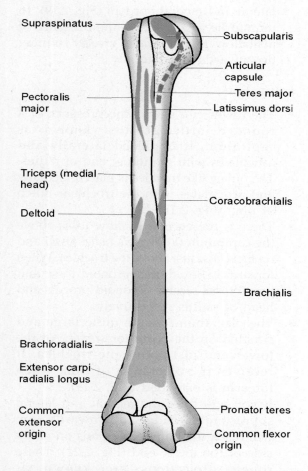

Fig. 2.22: Attachment of the muscles on the anterior aspect of right humerus

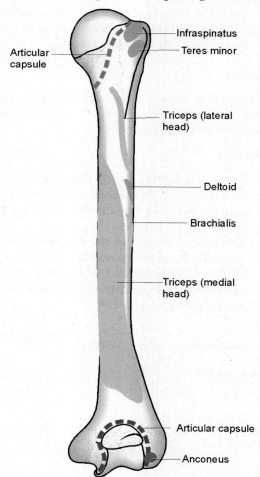

Fig. 2.23: Attachment of muscles on posterior aspect of right humerus

Shaft

Anterior Aspect

- On the anterior aspect of shaft, the medial lip of bicipital groove gives attachment to *teres major* while lateral lip to the *pectoralis major*. The floor of the bicipital groove gives insertion to *latissimus dorsi* (Fig. 2.22).
- On the V shaped deltoid tuberosity *deltoids* is attached.
- The *coracobrachialis* is attached on the middle of medial border.
- The *brachialis* muscle arises from the front aspect of lower half of shaft.
- The *pronator teres* takes origin from medial supracondylar ridge.
- The lateral supracondylar ridge gives origin to *brachioradialis* and *extensor carpi radialis longus*.

Posterior Aspect

- *Lateral head of triceps* arises above the radial groove (Fig. 2.23).
- Below the radial groove, the posterior surface gives origin to the *medial head of triceps*.

Lower End

- The front of medial epicondyle gives origin to *superficial flexor muscles* of forearm. This origin is known as "common flexor origin".
- The anterior aspect of lateral epicondyle gives origin to *extensors* of forearm hence known as "common extensor origin".
- The *anconeus* originates from the posterior surface of the lateral epicondyle.

Ligaments Attached to Bone

- The attachments of *articular capsule* for shoulder joint and elbow joints are shown in Figs. 2.22 and 2.23.

- The *ulnar collateral ligament* of elbow joint is attached to the medial epicondyle.
- The *radial collateral ligament* is attached to the lateral epicondyle.

Nerves and Vessels Related to the Bone

- The surgical neck of the humerus is related to the anterior and posterior *circumflex humeral vessels* and to the *axillary nerve* (Fig. 2.24).

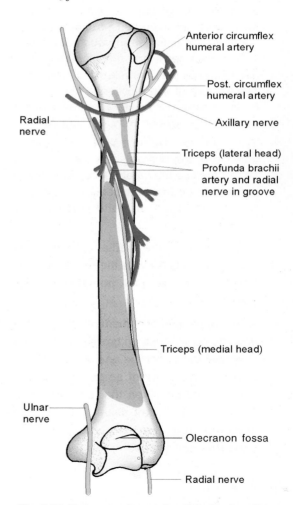

Fig. 2.24: Nerves and vessels related to humerus

- The radial nerve and *profunda/brachii* vessels are related to the radial groove.
- The *ulnar nerve* lies just posterior to the medial epicondyle.

CLINICAL IMPORTANCE

- The common sites of fracture are surgical neck, middle of the shaft and supracondylar region. The fracture of surgical neck of humerus is common in old people. The axillary nerve, which is in direct contact of neck, may get injured. The supracondylar fractures are common in young individual. The median nerve and brachial artery may get injured as they are related to lower end. The fracture of middle of shaft may be due to direct blow to arm. Here the radial nerve in the radial groove may get injured.

- The avulsion fractures of the greater tubercle of the humerus are also common (in this fracture the greater tubercle is pulled away from the rest of upper end). This may result due to fall on hand while arm is abducted.

- The fracture of the medial epicondyle is usually associated with the injury of ulnar nerve, as it lies just posterior to the epicondyle.

- As the upper end of humerus is the growing end, the bone keeps on growing in a young individual even after the amputation of arm. Hence, at the time of amputation of arm care should be taken that sufficient soft tissue should be left distal to the site of amputation so the bony stump will not penetrate soft tissues.

Ossification

The upper end ossifies by 3 and lower end by 4 secondary centers (Fig. 2.25).

Upper end is the growing end as the secondary centre appears first and fuses last (at 20 years).

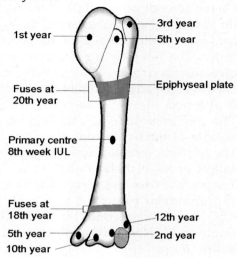

Fig. 2.25: Ossification of humerus

RADIUS

The radius is situated on the lateral side (thumb side) of the forearm. Like any other long bone it also consists of upper end, shaft and lower end (Figs. 2.26 and 2.27). The upper (proximal) end of radius is narrow while its lower end is wide. The upper end presents a disc shaped head, a neck and medially directed radial tuberosity. The shaft of the radius has a laterally directed convexity. The medial border is sharp and called as interosseous border. The lower end is wide and shows anterior, posterior, medial and lateral surfaces. The posterior surface of the lower end is rough and presents a dorsal tubercle. A projection (styloid process) is present on the lateral aspect of the lower end.

Side Determination

- Keep the bone vertically in such a way that

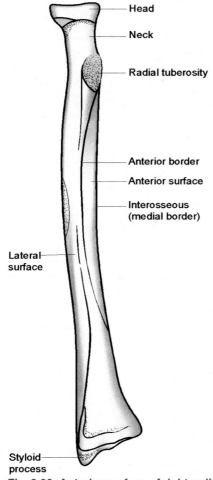

Fig. 2.26: Anterior surface of right radius

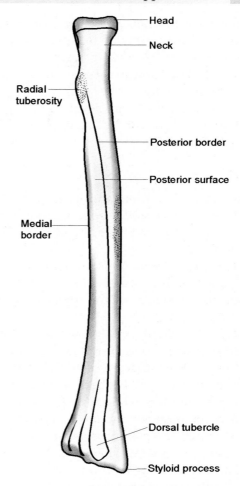

Fig. 2.27: Posterior surface of right radius

narrow disc shaped upper end is directed upward (proximally).

- At the expanded lower end, the dorsal tubercle should face backward and styloid process directed laterally and downwards.

- In this position, a sharp border of the shaft (interosseous border) should be directed medially.

Anatomical Position

Hold the bone vertically in such a way that the head is directed upwards, radial tuberosity and sharp border medially, and dorsal tubercle posteriorly.

General Features

Upper End

The upper end consists of head, neck and radial tuberosity (Figs. 2.26 and 2.27).

- The disc shaped head shows an upper surface, which is slightly concave to articulate with the capitulum of humerus.

- The circumference of the head articulates medially with the radial notch of ulna to form *superior radioulnar joint*. The rest of the circumference of the head is surrounded by *annular ligament*.

- The constriction just below the head is known as neck.
- There is a prominent elevation just below the medial part of neck. This is known as *radial tuberosity*

Shaft

Shaft shows 3 borders and three surfaces.

- Trace *anterior border* from anterior aspect of radial tuberosity to the *styloid process* (Fig. 2.26).
- Trace the *posterior border* from the posterior aspect of the radial tuberosity to the posterior aspect of the lower end (Fig. 2.27).
- Trace the sharp *medial (interosseous) border* from lower aspect of radial tuberosity to the posterior margin of *ulnar notch*.
- The *anterior surface* lies between anterior and medial borders while *posterior surface* lies between posterior and medial borders. The *lateral surface* is present between anterior and posterior borders. This surface is convex laterally and shows a rough area near the middle part of the shaft.

Lower End

The lower end is the expanded end and shows anterior, posterior, lateral and medial surfaces.

- It also shows an inferior surface, which is smooth (articular) and articulates with scaphoid laterally and lunate bone medially to form the wrist joint (Fig. 2.28).
- The lateral surface when traced downwards, projects as styloid process.
- The medial surface shows ulnar notch. It articulates with the head of ulna to form *inferior radioulnar joint*.

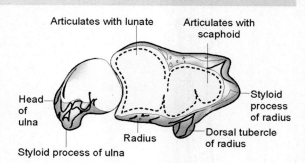

Fig. 2.28: The inferior surface of radius and ulna of right side

Particular Features

Muscles Attached to the Radius

Upper End

- The *biceps brachii* is inserted on the rough posterior part of the radial tuberosity (Fig. 2.29). The anterior smooth part of the radial tuberosity is in relation with the *bursa*.

Shaft and Lower End

- The upper part of the anterior border gives origin to the radial head of *flexor digitorum superficialis*.
- The upper 2/3 of the anterior surface gives origin to the *flexor pollicis longus*.
- The *pronator quadratus* is inserted into lowermost part of anterior surface. The attachment also extends on the medial surface of lower end.
- The upper part of the lateral, anterior and posterior surfaces gives insertion to *supinator* (Figs. 2.29 and 2.30).
- The rough area on the middle of the lateral surface gives insertion to *pronator teres*.
- The muscle *brachioradialis* is inserted into the lowest part of lateral surface just above the styloid process.
- The *abductor pollicis longus* and *extensor pollicis brevis* arise from the posterior surface of the shaft.

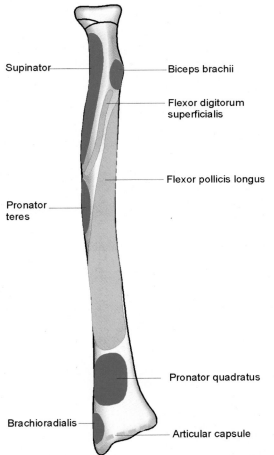

Fig. 2.29: Attachment of the muscles on the anterior aspects of the radius

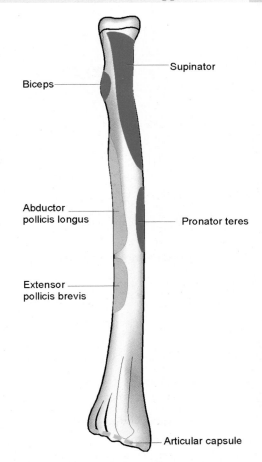

Fig. 2.30: Attachment of the muscles on the posterior aspects of the radius

Ligaments Attached to the Bone

- Note the attachment of the *articular capsule* of wrist joint on the lower end of the radius (Figs. 2.29 and 2.30).
- The *interosseous membrane* is attached to lower ¾ of medial border.
- The *articular disc* of the inferior radioulnar joint is attached to the lower border of the ulnar notch.
- The anterior border near the lower end gives attachment to the *extensor retinaculum.*

- The *radial collateral ligament* of wrist joint is attached to the tip of the styloid process (Fig. 2.31).

Tendons and Arteries in Relation to the Bone

- The relationship of tendons on the dorsal aspect of the lower end is shown in Fig. 2.32.
- The radial artery is related to the anterior surface of lower end. Here the pulsations of artery can be easily felt by applying pressure against the radial bone Fig. 2.31.

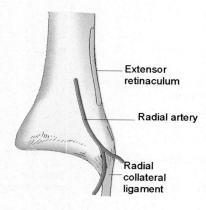

Fig. 2.31: Attachment of ligaments and relation of radial artery on ventral aspect

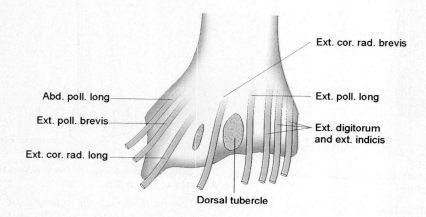

Fig. 2.32: Tendons related to dorsal aspect of lower end

CLINICAL IMPORTANCE

Though the fracture of radius may occur at its upper end and shaft but the fracture of the distal end of radius is most common especially in old women. Fracture of the lower end of the radius is called as Colles's fracture. The fracture usually results due to fall on outstretched hand. The distal fragment overrides and is displaced dorsally (Fig. 2.33). This results into shortening of radius. As a result the styloid process of both the bones (radius and ulna) now lie almost at the same level. The clinical deformity is often referred to as "dinner fork deformity".

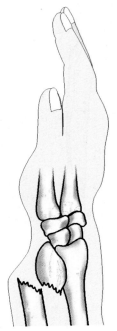

Fig. 2.33: Colles's fracture. Note the overriding of distal fragment of radius

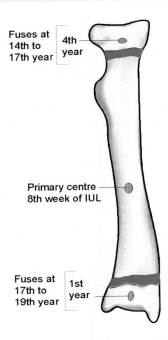

Fuses at 14th to 17th year | 4th year

Primary centre 8th week of IUL

Fuses at 17th to 19th year | 1st year

Fig. 2.34: Ossification of radius

Ossification

Radius ossifies by one primary and two secondary centers, i.e., one for each end (Fig. 2.34). Lower end is the growing end.

ULNA

Ulna is the medial bone of forearm. It is longer than the radius. Ulna has an upper end, a lower end and a shaft (Figs. 2.35 and 2.36). The upper end of ulna is expanded, irregular and presents a deep notch, which faces anteriorly. This notch is called as *trochlear notch* and it articulates with the trochlea of humerus at the elbow joint. While its lower end is small and has a tiny styloid process. You should remember that the lower end of ulna is called as head. The shaft has a sharp lateral margin. This margin gives attachment to the broad, flat, fibrous connective tissue called interosseous membrane. Ulna is connected with the radius by interosseous membrane.

Side Determination

- Hold the bone vertically in such a way that its expanded hook like end is directed upwards and small rounded lower end directed downwards.
- The concavity of trochlear notch (at the upper end) should face anteriorly.
- The sharp border of the shaft should be directed laterally.

Anatomical Position

Hold the bone vertically in such a way that the trochlear notch faces anteriorly, sharp border of the shaft laterally, and styloid process at the lower end is present posteriorly.

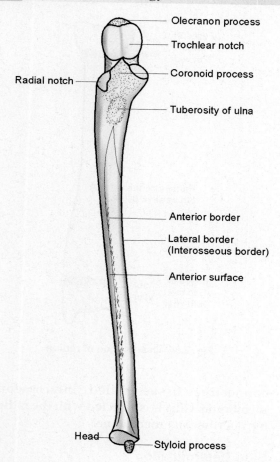

Fig. 2.35: Anterior aspect of the right ulna

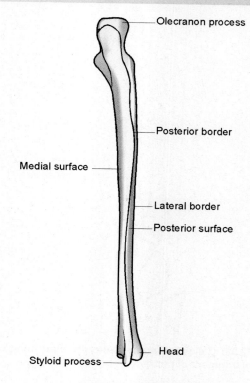

Fig. 2.36: Posterior aspect of right ulna

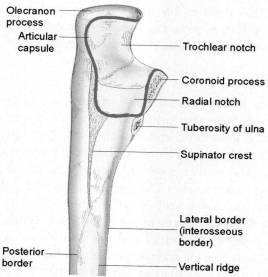

Fig. 2.37: The upper end of right ulna showing olecranon and coronoid processes

General Features

Upper End

The upper end of the ulna presents *olecranon* process, *coronoid* processes and two articular surfaces, i.e., *trochlear* and *radial notches* (Fig. 2.37).

Olecranon Process

- The olecranon process is the uppermost part of the ulna (Fig. 2.37). It has superior, anterior, posterior, medial and lateral surfaces.

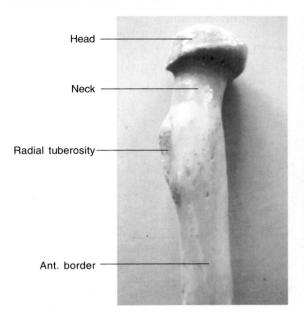

Head

Neck

Radial tuberosity

Ant. border

Fig. 2G: Upper end of left radius, ant. view

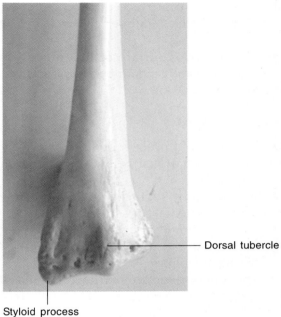

Dorsal tubercle

Styloid process

Fig. 2H: Posterior view, lower end radius

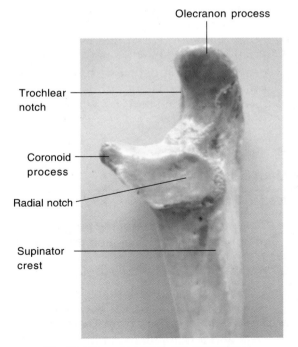

Olecranon process

Trochlear notch

Coronoid process

Radial notch

Supinator crest

Fig. 2I: Ulna upper end, lateral surface

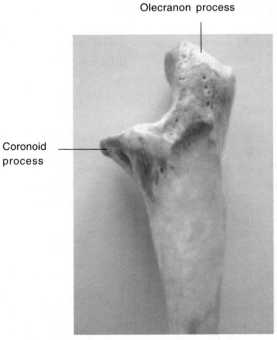

Olecranon process

Coronoid process

Fig. 2J: Ulna upper end, medial surface

- The anterior surface of the olecranon process forms the upper part of trochlear notch.
- The posterior surface of this process is triangular and smooth because it lies just beneath the skin.

Coronoid Process

- The coronoid process projects anteriorly from the shaft just below the olecranon (Fig. 2.37).
- It has four surfaces, i.e., superior, anterior, medial and lateral.
- The superior (upper) surface is almost horizontal and forms the lower part of trochlear notch.
- The anterior surface is triangular and is rough in its lower part. The rough area is known as *tuberosity of ulna*.

Radial Notch

- The lateral surface of the coronoid process has a concave articular area (Fig. 2.37). This is known as radial notch. It articulates with the head of radius forming the *superior radioulnar joint*.

Trochlear Notch

- It articulates with the trochlea of humerus. It is formed by the anterior surface of olecranon and upper surface of coronoid process (Fig. 2.37). There may be a non-articular area (groove) between the two parts.

Lower End

- The lower end (head) is small and rounded.
- Anteriorly and laterally it articulates with ulnar notch of the radius to form inferior radioulnar joint.

- The inferior surface is separated from the cavity of wrist joint by an articular disc.
- The styloid process projects downwards from the posteromedial aspect of the lower end.

Shaft

- The cross-section of shaft is almost triangular in shape.
- It presents anterior, lateral and posterior borders and anterior, medial and posterior surfaces.
- The lateral or *interosseous border* is sharp. When traced upwards, it becomes continuous with a rough ridge present just posterior to radial notch. This rough ridge is known as *supinator crest* (Fig. 2.37).
- Anterior and posterior borders are rounded. The anterior border begins at the lower end of tuberosity of ulna and ends on the anterior aspect of *styloid process*.
- Anterior surface lies between anterior and interosseous border and shows the presence of an oblique ridge in its lower part.
- Posterior surface lies between interosseous and posterior border. The posterior surface is subdivided into medial and lateral parts by a vertical ridge (Fig. 2.37).

Particular Features

Muscles Attached to Bone

Upper End

- The *triceps* is inserted on the posterior part of upper surface of olecranon process (Fig. 2.39).
- *Brachialis* is attached on the anterior surface of coronoid process and the tuberosity of the ulna (Fig. 2.38).
- *The supinator* arises from the supinator crest and a triangular area just below the radial notch.

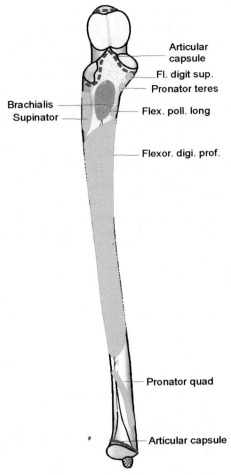

Fig. 2.38: Attachment of muscles on the anterior surface of right ulna

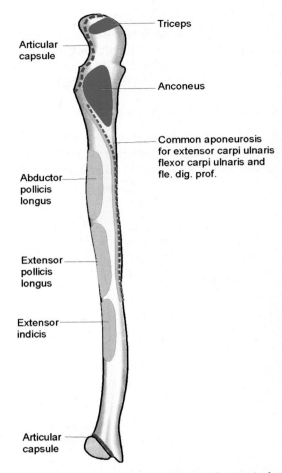

Fig. 2.39: Attachment of muscles on the posterior surface of left ulna

- The medial border of coronoid process gives origin to the ulnar head of *flexor digitorum superficialis* above and *pronator teres* below.
- The *anconeus* is inserted into the lateral aspect of the olecranon and upper part of the posterior surface of the shaft (Fig. 2.39).
- The ulnar head of the pronator teres arises from the medial margin of the coronoid process.

- The ulnar head of the *flexor carpi ulnaris* arises from the medial side of olecranon process and from the upper two third of posterior border through an aponeurosis. From the same aponeurosis, ulnar head of *extensor carpi ulnaris* also arises (Fig. 2.39).

Shaft

- *Flexor digitorum profundus* takes origin from the anterior and medial surface of shaft.
- On the anterior surface the oblique ridge gives origin to *pronator quadratus*.

- Three muscles are attached on posterior surface (between interosseous border and a vertical ridge) from above downwards i.e., *abductor pollicis longus*, *extensor pollicis longus* and *extensor indices* (Fig. 2.39).

Ligaments Attached to Bone

- The *capsular ligament* of the elbow joint is attached to the margins of the coronoid and olecranon process (Figs. 2.38 and 2.39).

- The capsular ligament of the inferior radioulnar joint is attached close to the articular area (Fig. 2.38 and 2.39).
- The apex of triangular articular disc is attached to the lateral aspect of the styloid process.
- The interosseous membrane is attached to the sharp interosseous border (Fig. 2.40).
- The *annular ligament* of superior radio-ulnar joint is attached to the anterior and posterior border of radial notch.
- The *oblique cord* is attached on the lateral aspect of the ulnar tuberosity.
- The *ulnar collateral ligament* of wrist joint is attached to the tip of styloid process.

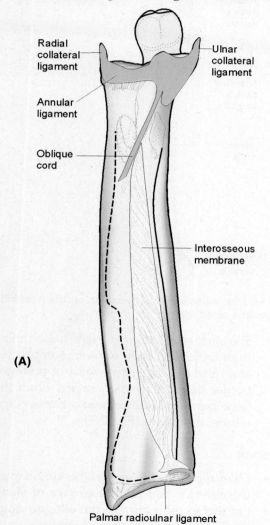

(A)

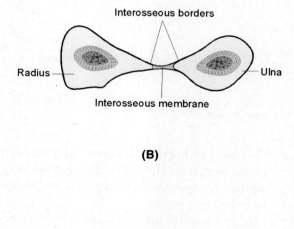

(B)

Fig. 2.40: (A) Attachment of interosseous membrane, (B) Transverse section through radius and ulna

CLINICAL IMPORTANCE

Though the fractures of both the radius and ulna may result due to severe injury but isolated fracture of radius and ulna may also occur. The most common fracture of ulna along with radius is through the middle of shaft or at its lower end. Sometimes the fracture of the olecranon can occur due to fall on elbow.

Ossification

Ulna ossifies by 3 centers, i.e., one primary and two secondary, i.e., one each for upper and lower end (Fig. 2.41). Lower end is the growing end.

BONES OF THE HAND

Bones of the hand consists of *carpals*, *metacarpals* and *phalanges* (Fig. 2.42).

Carpal Bones

The skeleton of the wrist consists of eight small bones (Fig. 2.43), which are arranged in two transverse rows of four bones each. These bones are called *carpal bones*. They are named as per their shapes.

The proximal row, from lateral to medial side, consists of:

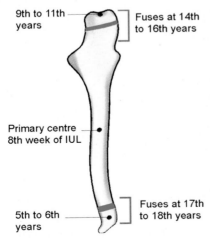

Fig. 2.41: Ossification of ulna

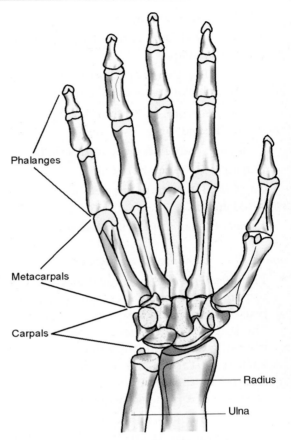

Fig. 2.42: Bones of the right hand

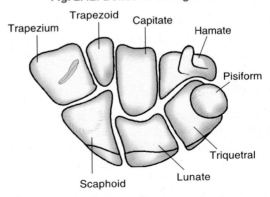

Fig. 2.43: Schematic diagram of left carpal bones as seen from anterior aspect

Scaphoid (It is a boat shaped bone and has a prominent tubercle on its anterior aspect).

Lunate (It is moon shaped).

Triquetrum (It has three corners and is pyramidal in shape).

Pisiform (It is pea shaped small bone that lies on the anterior surface of the triquetrum).

The carpal bones in distal row, from lateral to medial, are:

Trapezium (table shaped, four sided).

Trapezoid (wedge shaped).

Capitate (It is cap shaped and has a rounded head).

Hamate (It has a hook shaped process).

Joints Formed by the Carpal Bones

- The *wrist joint* is formed between the proximal surfaces of three carpal bones of proximal row and lower end of radius. The scaphoid and lunate of the proximal row articulates with the inferior articular surface of radius, while triquetrum is related to the articular disc and thus separated from head of ulna.

- Carpal bones are joined to one another by interosseous ligaments and *intercarpal joints*.

- The distal articular surfaces of the carpal bones of distal row articulate with the metacarpals to form *carpometacarpal joints*.

CLINICAL IMPORTANCE

The common injury of the wrist consists of fracture of the scaphoid or lunate.

- The fracture of the scaphoid is most common. It results due to a fall on outstretched hand. In this condition, the line of fracture passes almost from the middle of bone dividing the bone into proximal and distal fragments. Patient complains of pain in the scaphoid fossa (lateral side of wrist).

- As the nutrient arteries of scaphoid enter the distal end of the bone, the proximal segment is devoid of the blood supply after fracture. This may results into avascular necrosis (death due to inadequate blood supply) of the proximal fragment of the scaphoid. Thus scaphoid fracture heals poorly, i.e., may take several months to heal.

- The fracture of hamate also heals poorly due to the traction produced by the attached muscles. As the ulnar nerve lies close to the hook of hamate, it may also get injured due to the fracture of hamate.

Metacarpals

Metacarpals are miniature long bones, which form the skeleton of palm (Fig. 2.42). They are five in number and are numbered from lateral to the medial side. The metacarpal of thumb is known as first (I) metacarpal while that of little finger is known as fifth (V) metacarpal.

- Each metacarpal bone consists of proximal base, intermediate shaft and a distal head (Fig. 2.44).

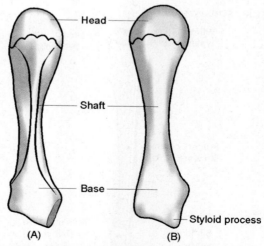

Fig. 2.44: General features of a metacarpal bone (A) Ventral (palmar) surface (B) Dorsal surface

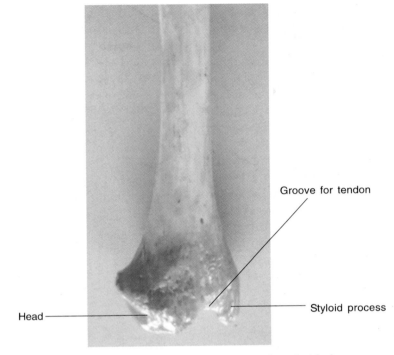

Groove for tendon

Styloid process

Head

Fig. 2K: Lower end of left ulna, as seen from behind

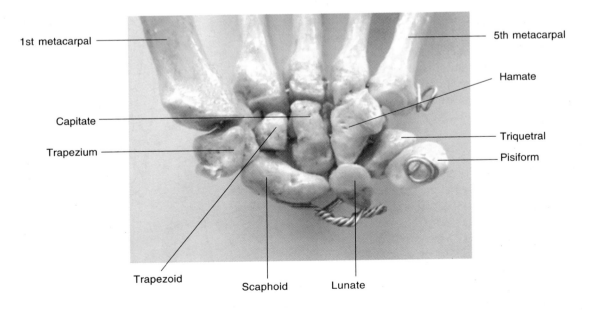

1st metacarpal

5th metacarpal

Hamate

Capitate

Triquetral

Trapezium

Pisiform

Trapezoid   Scaphoid   Lunate

Fig. 2L: Ventral aspect of left carpal bones and base of metacarpals

- The proximal ends or bases of metacarpals are irregularly expanded and articulate with the carpal bones.
- The distal ends (heads) are rounded and articulate with the proximal phalanges.
- The shaft of each metacarpal is curved with the concavity looking forwards. It has three surfaces, i.e., medial, lateral and posterior.
- The first metacarpal is easily distinguished from the rest because it is thickest and shortest of all the metacarpals. The articular surface at its base is concavo-convex which articulates with trapezium. Third metacarpal can also be differentiated from the rest because it has a styloid process on the lateral side of its base.

Joints Formed by the Metacarpals

- The distal articular surfaces of the carpal bones of distal row articulate with the metacarpals to form *carpometacarpal joints*. The trapezium articulates with the first metacarpal, trapezoid with second, capitate with third and hamate with fourth and fifth metacarpals.
- The distal articular surfaces of metacarpals articulate with the proximal articular surfaces of proximal phalanges to form *carpometacarpal joints*.

Phalanges

Phalanges are the bones of digits. Each digit has three phalanges (i.e., proximal, middle and distal) except first (for thumb), which has only two phalanges (Fig. 2.42).

Each phalanx has a proximal base, a body and a distal head. The proximal phalanges are longest and articulate with the head of metacarpals at their bases to form metacarpophalangeal joints. The middle phalanges are intermediate in size and articulate at their

bases with the heads of proximal phalanges to form proximal interphalangeal joints. The distal phalanges are smallest, flattened and expanded at their distal ends (non-articular) to form the nail beds.

Particular Features of the Bones of Hand

Insertion of forearm muscles on the palmar surface of hand (Fig. 2.45).

- The *flexor carpi ulnaris* is attached on the pisiform bone. From this bone *abductor digiti minimi* also takes origin.

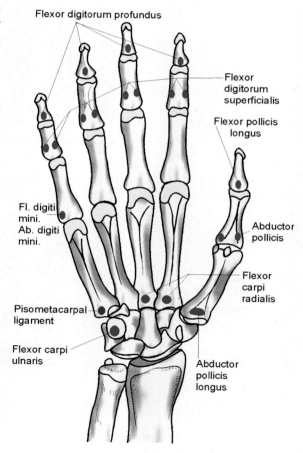

Fig. 2.45: Attachment (insertion) of forearm muscles on the palmar surface of right hand

- *Flexor carpi radialis* is inserted on the base of 2nd and 3rd metacarpals on their palmar surface.
- The *flexor digitorum profundus* is inserted on the bases of distal phalanges, while *flexor digitorum superficialis* is inserted on both the sides of middle phalanges of all the fingers except that of thumb.
- The *flexor pollicis longus* is inserted on the base of the distal phalanx of thumb, on its palmar surface.

Insertion of forearm muscles on dorsal aspect of hand and dorsal interossei are shown in Fig. 2.46.

- The *extensor carpi ulnaris* is attached to the base of fifth metacarpal; *abductor pollicis longus* to the base of first; *extensor carpi radialis longus* to the base of second; *extensor carpi radialis brevis* to the bases of 2nd and 3rd metacarpals.

- The *extensor pollicis brevis* is attached on the base of proximal phalanx, while *extensor pollicis longus* to the base of distal phalanx of thumb.
- The *extensor digitorum* is inserted on the base of middle and distal phalanges of all the fingers except thumb.
- The origin and insertion of *dorsal interossei* is also seen in this figure.

The origin and insertion of the *thenar*, *hypothenar* and *palmer interossei* are shown in Fig. 2.47.

Attachments of Ligaments

- The attachment of carpal bones with each other (due to their shape) presents a concavity forward. The attachment of *flexor retinaculum* medially to the hook of hamate and pisiform bone and laterally

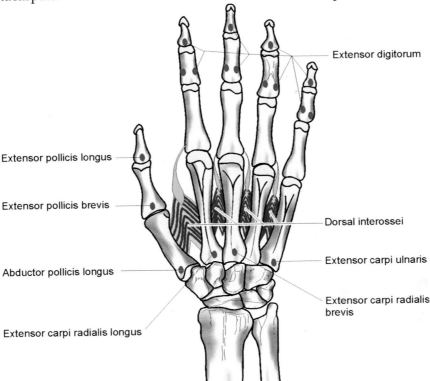

Fig. 2.46: Attachment of muscles on the dorsal surface of right hand

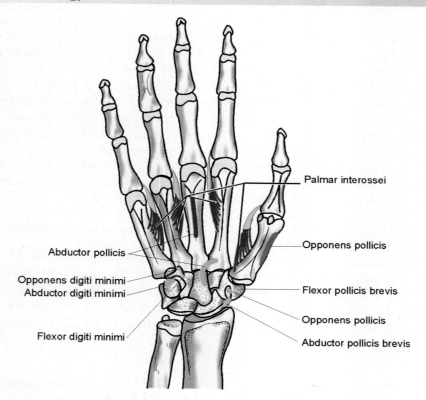

Fig. 2.47: Attachment of muscles on palmar surface of right hand

to the tubercles of scaphoid and trapezium forms an osteofascial *carpal tunnel*. Through this tunnel passes the tendons, vessels and nerve from forearm to hand.

- Pisiform bone gives attachment to two ligaments (Fig. 2.48), i.e., first extending from pisiform to the base of fifth metacarpal (*pisometacarpal*) and second from pisiform to the hook of hamate (*pisohamate*).
- The medial end of the *extensor retinaculum* is attached to the triquetral and pisiform bones.
- The lateral margins of each phalanx give attachment to *fibrous flexor sheath*.

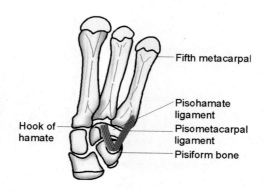

Fig. 2.48: Attachment of pisometacarpal and pisohamate ligaments

Ossification (Fig. 2.49)

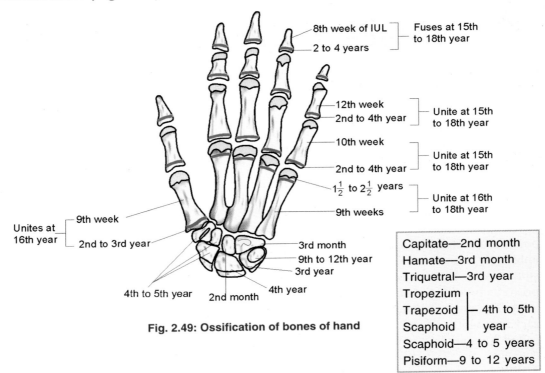

Fig. 2.49: Ossification of bones of hand

8th week of IUL
2 to 4 years
Fuses at 15th to 18th year

12th week
2nd to 4th year
Unite at 15th to 18th year

10th week
2nd to 4th year
Unite at 15th to 18th year

$1\frac{1}{2}$ to $2\frac{1}{2}$ years
9th weeks
Unite at 16th to 18th year

Unites at 16th year
9th week
2nd to 3rd year

3rd month
9th to 12th year
3rd year

4th to 5th year   2nd month   4th year

Capitate—2nd month
Hamate—3rd month
Triquetral—3rd year
Tropezium
Trapezoid   4th to 5th
Scaphoid   year
Scaphoid—4 to 5 years
Pisiform—9 to 12 years

3 Bones of the Lower Limb

The lower limb consists of many regions (Fig. 3.1). Following bones are present in various regions of the lower limb:

Pelvic (Hip) Region

Bones of this region form pelvic girdle. The pelvic girdle consists of two hip bones. These bones are united to each other in the midline anteriorly to form a joint known as the *pubic symphysis*. Both the hip bones unite posteriorly with the sacrum at the sacroiliac joint. The pelvic girdle (two hip bones) and sacrum together form a basin like structure called *bony pelvis*.

Thigh

This region consists of a single bone called as femur. The upper end of this bone articulates with hip bone to form *hip joint*. The lower end of femur articulates with the upper end of tibia to form knee joint.

Leg

This region consists of two long bones, i.e., medially placed tibia and laterally placed fibula. These two bones, at their lower end, articulate with talus to form *ankle joint*.

Foot

The skeleton of foot consists of many bones, i.e., tarsals, metatarsals and phalanges. These bones form many joints, i.e., *intertarsal, tarsometatarsal, metatarsophalangeal and interphalangeal*.

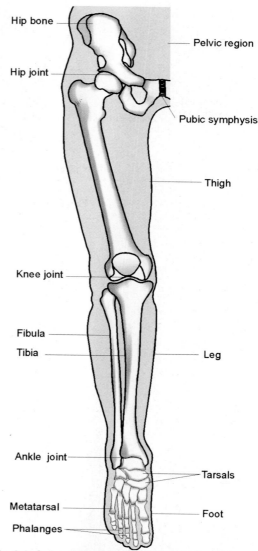

Fig. 3.1: Schematic diagram showing bones of lower limb

HIP BONE

The hip bone is a large, irregular and flat bone. The middle portion of the bone is constricted and carries a cup shaped deep cavity on the lateral aspect of the bone. This cavity is known as *acetabulum* (Fig. 3.2). The bone is expanded above and below the acetabulum. There is presence of a large oval or triangular aperture just below and medial to the acetabulum. It is called as *obturator foramen*. The bone above the acetabulum is expanded and flat. This portion is called as *ilium*. The bone below the acetabulum consists of two parts, i.e., the anterior and inferior, *pubis* and posterior and inferior, *ischium.*

(Though an adult hip bone is a single bone but at birth each hip bone consists of three separate primary bones, i.e., ilium, ischium and pubis. These three bones are joined to each other by a Y shaped tri-radiate hyaline cartilage. These three components of hip bones join each other at acetabulum (Fig. 3.3). However, these three bones begin to fuse with each other at 15 to 17 years of age.

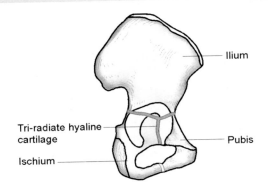

Fig. 3.3: In a young hip bone tri-radiate cartilage separates three parts of right hip bone

Though in an adult bone the site of fusion is not visible between three bones, their names are still used as three parts of hip bone). In Fig. 3.4 medial view of hip bone is shown.

Side Determination

Take the help of your teacher to determine the side of hip bone.

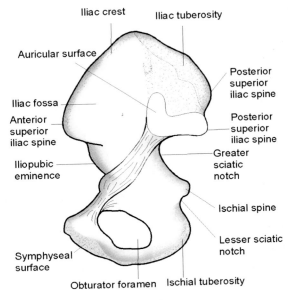

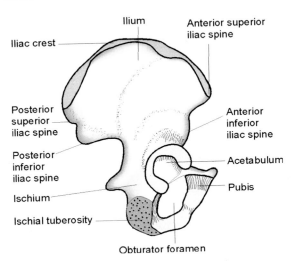

Fig. 3.2: Lateral view of the right hip bone

Fig. 3.4: Medial view of right hip bone

- The expanded flat part called as ilium, should be kept upwards (superiorly).
- The other expanded part (pubis and ischium) with the obturator foramen should be kept downwards (inferiorly).
- The acetabulum should face laterally.
- The lower expanded part (below acetabulum) has two parts, i.e., thin pubis and thick ischium. The pubis should be directed anteriorly and ischium posteriorly.

Many students find it difficult to keep the bone in anatomical position. Therefore you should learn the anatomical position of this bone only after you have learnt the general features of all the three parts (ilium, ischium and pubis).

ILIUM

Ilium is the largest part of hip bone (Figs. 3.2 and 3.4). It forms the upper fan shaped expanded part above the acetabulum. The upper 2/5th of the acetabulum is formed by the ilium.

General Features

The ilium presents:
- *Two ends*–Upper and lower.
- *Three borders*–Anterior, posterior and medial.
- *Three surfaces*–Gluteal (lateral), iliac fossa and sacropelvic.

Ends

Upper end–The upper end is in the form of an expanded border. It is also called as *iliac crest*. The iliac crest is thick and curved border, which is convex upwards. This extends between two projections, i.e., *anterior superior iliac spine* and *posterior superior iliac* spine.

- The iliac crest is subdivided into *ventral* and *dorsal segments*. The ventral segment is anterior 2/3rd of the iliac crest and presents an outward convexity, while dorsal segment forms posterior 1/3 of the crest and presents outward concavity.
- The thick ventral segment of the iliac crest shows an *outer lip, intermediate area* and *inner lip*.
- The outer lip presents a prominence about 5 cm behind the anterior superior iliac spine. This is called as *tubercle of the iliac crest*.
- The dorsal segment of the iliac crest presents medial and lateral sloping surfaces separated by a ridge.

Lower end–The lower end of ilium lies in the acetabulum and forms the upper 2/5th of this cup shaped cavity. At the lower end, ilium becomes continuous with the ischium and pubis. The lower end of ilium meets with the pubis at *iliopubic eminence.*

Borders

Anterior border–The anterior border of the ilium extends from anterior superior iliac spine to the acetabulum. The lowest part of this border projects forwards, near the upper margin of the acetabulum, to form anterior inferior iliac spine.

Posterior border–This extends from the posterior superior iliac spine to the greater sciatic notch. Here it becomes continuous with the upper end of the posterior border of the ischium. This border presents posterior inferior iliac spine and greater sciatic notch.

Medial border–The medial border is present on the inner aspect (medial surface) of the ilium. This border extends from iliac crest to the iliopubic eminence. It lies between iliac fossa and sacropelvic surface of ilium. The medial border is rough in its upper 1/3rd, sharp in its middle third and rounded in lower 1/3rd. The lower one third of medial border is called as *arcuate line*.

Surfaces

The ilium has an outer *gluteal surface* (Fig. 3.2) and an inner surface, which is further divided into *iliac fossa* and *sacropelvic surface* (Fig. 3.4).

Gluteal surface–This surface is the lateral surface (outer aspect) of the ilium. It has three rough curved lines (the posterior, anterior and inferior gluteal lines), which divide the gluteal surface into four areas.

Iliac fossa–The iliac fossa is present on the anterior part of the medial surface of the ilium, in front of the medial border. Iliac fossa presents shallow concavity and has smooth surface.

Sacropelvic surface–This surface is also present on the medial surface of ilium behind the iliac fossa and medial border. It is subdivided into three parts, i.e., *iliac tuberosity, auricular surface* and *pelvic surface*.
- The iliac tuberosity is upper rough part.
- The auricular surface is the ear shaped and articular in nature. It is the middle part of the sacropelvic surface, which articulates with the sacrum to form the *sacroiliac joint*.
- The pelvic surface is smooth surface below and in front of the auricular surface. This surface is continuous with the pelvic surface of the ischium. This surface may present a *pre-auricular sulcus* in the females who have given birth to children (multiparous).

PUBIS

The pubis or pubic bone is situated ventro-medial to ilium and ischium. It consists of *body*, a *superior ramus* and an *inferior ramus*.

Body of Pubis

The body is flattened and presents three surfaces, i.e., anterior, posterior (pelvic) and medial (*symphyseal*). The anterior surface faces downwards, forwards and laterally. Posterior surface is smooth and directed upwards and backwards. The symphyseal surface articulates with the corresponding surface of the opposite pubic bone to form a joint known as *pubic symphysis*. This surface show the presence of ridges that change with increasing age (*See* Further Details).

The superior border of the body of pubis is thick and known as *pubic crest*. At the lateral end of pubic crest there is a projection, the *pubic tubercle*.

Superior Ramus of Pubis

The superior ramus of pubis arises from the upper and lateral part of the body of pubis. Laterally it extends above the obturator foramen upto the iliopubic eminence where it joins the ilium. Here it also forms the pubic part (anterior 1/5) of acetabulum. It has three borders (anterior, posterior and inferior) and three surfaces (pectineal, pelvic and obturator).

Borders

- The *anterior border* is also known as obturator crest and extends from pubic tubercle to the acetabular notch.
- The *posterior border* or pectineal line (pecten pubis) extends from pubic tubercle to the iliopubic eminence. It is a sharp border, which behind the iliopubic eminence becomes continuous with the arcuate line of ilium.

- The *inferior border* forms the upper border of obturator foramen.

Surfaces

- The *pectineal surface* is situated between pectineal line and obturator crest. It is triangular in shape and extends between pubic tubercle and iliopubic eminence.
- The *pelvic surface* lies between pectineal and inferior border of superior ramus. It is smooth and continuous medially with the pelvic surface of the body of pubis.
- The *obturator surface* is situated between obturator crest and inferior border. It is a grooved surface and forms the upper boundary of obturator canal.

Inferior Ramus of Pubis

It extends downwards and laterally from the lower and lateral part of the body of pubis. The inferior ramus of pubis meets the ramus of ischium to form the *conjoined ischiopubic rami*. The conjoined ischiopubic rami forms medial boundary of obtutrator foramen. It has an anterior and a posterior surface.

ISCHIUM

The ischium forms the posteroinferior part of the hip bone. It consists of a body and a ramus.

Body

Body lies posteroinferior to the acetabulum. It has two ends (upper and lower), three borders (anterior, posterior and lateral) and three surfaces (femoral, dorsal and pelvic).

Ends

- The *upper end* of body forms the 2/5 of posteiror and inferior part of the acetabulum.

- The *lower end* forms the *ischial tuberosity*. The ramus of the ischium extends from the lower end of the body upwards, forwards and medially to meet the inferior ramus of the pubis.

Borders

- The *anterior border* forms the posterior margin of obturator foramen.
- The *posterior border* is continuous with the posterior border of ilium. It presents a triangular projection called as ischial spine. The ischial spine is placed between the greater sciatic notch (above) and lesser sciatic notch (below).
- The *lateral border* extends from lower margin of the acetabulum and becomes continuous with the lateral margin of ischial tuberosity.

Surfaces

- The *femoral surface* is situated between anterior and lateral borders.
- The *dorsal surface* is continuous above with the gluteal surface of ilium. The lower part of dorsal surface has a large rough area known as *ischial tuberosity* (Fig. 3.5).

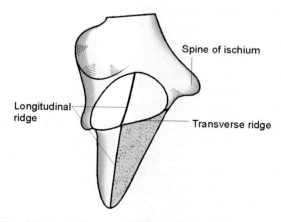

Spine of ischium

Longitudinal ridge

Transverse ridge

Fig. 3.5: Schematic diagram showing the ischial tuberosity

- This tuberosity is divided by a transverse ridge in an upper quadrilateral part and a lower triangular part. Each of these parts (upper and lower) is again divided into medial land lateral parts.
- The *pelvic surface* of ischium is smooth and lies between anterior and posterior borders.

Ramus of Ischium

It extends from the lower part of body and runs upwards, forwards and medially. Here it meets the inferior ramus of the pubis and forms the *conjoined ischiopubic ramus*. The conjoined ischiopubic ramus presents upper and lower borders and an outer and inner surface (Figs. 3.2 and 3.4).

Obturator Foramen

It is a large triangular or oval foramen in the lower part of hip bone. It is situated between pubis and ischium. The obturator foramen is bounded above by the superior ramus of pubis, medially by body of pubis and conjoined ischiopubic ramus and laterally by the body of ischium.

Acetabulum

- The acetabulum is a deep cup shaped cavity facing laterally and anterior-inferiorly. It is situated on the constricted middle part of the hip bone. All the three parts of hip bone (pubis, ischium and ilium) contribute in its formation (Fig. 3.2).
- The acetabulum articulates with the head of the femur to form *hip joint.*
- The margin of the acetabulum is sharp and deficient in the anteroinferior part. This gap in the margin is called as *acetabular notch.*
- The floor of the acetabulum has a horseshoe shaped articular surface (*lunate surface*) and a non-articular central *acetabular fossa.*

Anatomical Position of Hip Bone

Keep the bone in such a way that:
- The pubic bone lies anteriorly and the symphyseal surface of pubis lies in the median plane.
- The acetabulum faces laterally and slightly anteriorly.
- The pubic tubercle and anterior superior iliac spine should lie in the same coronal plane.
- The posterior surface of the body of pubic bone should face postero-superiorly.
- The ischial spine and superior end of pubic symphysis are approximately in the same horizontal plane.

Particular Features

ILIUM

Attachment of Muscles on the Ventral 2/3rd of Iliac Crest (Fig. 3.6)

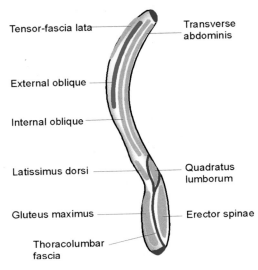

Tensor-fascia lata

Transverse abdominis

External oblique

Internal oblique

Latissimus dorsi

Quadratus lumborum

Gluteus maximus

Erector spinae

Thoracolumbar fascia

Fig. 3.6: Attachments on the left iliac crest

- The *external oblique muscle* of abdomen is inserted on the outer lip into the anterior 2/3rd of ventral segment of iliac crest.
- The *internal oblique* originates from the intermediate area of the ventral segment of iliac crest.
- The inner lip gives origin to *transverse abdominis*.
- The *tensor-fascia lata* muscle arises from the outer lip of iliac crest near its anterior part.
- Part of the *latissimus dorsi* arises from the posterior most part of the outer lip of ventral segment.
- The *quadratus lumborum* arises from the posterior one third of the inner lip of the ventral segment of the iliac crest.

Attachment of the Muscles on the Dorsal 1/3rd of the Iliac Crest (Fig. 3.6)

- The lateral surface of the dorsal segment of the iliac crest gives origin to the *gluteus maximus* muscle.
- The *erector spinae* arises from the medial surface of the dorsal segment of the iliac crest.

Attachment of the Muscles on the Outer Surface (Gluteal Surface) of Ilium (Fig. 3.7)

- The area behind posterior gluteal line gives origin to *gluteus maximus*.
- The area between anterior and inferior posterior gluteal lines gives origin to *gluteus medius*.
- The area between anterior and inferior lines gives origin to *gluteus minimus*.
- The area below the inferior gluteal line gives origin to the reflected head of rectus femoris.

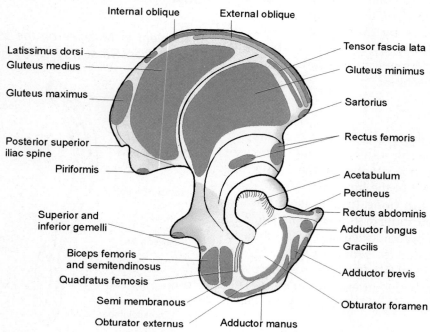

Fig. 3.7: Attachment of muscles on outer surface of right hip bone

Attachment of Muscles on the Inner Aspect (Sacropelvic Surface and Iliac Fossa) of the Ilium (Fig. 3.8)

- The *iliacus* muscle arises from the upper 2/3rd of the iliac fossa.
- The pelvic part of the sacropelvic surface of ilium above the obturator foramen gives origin to the *obturator internus* muscle.

Muscles Attached to the Anterior Border and Sciatic Notch of the Ilium

- The anterior superior iliac spine and an area below it gives origin to the *sartorius* muscle.
- The straight head of *rectus femoris* arises from the anterior inferior iliac spine.
- A small part of *piriformis* arises from the upper border of greater sciatic notch near the posterior inferior iliac spine.

PUBIS

Muscles Attached to the Pubic Bone

- The *adductor longus* muscle arises by a rounded tendon from the anterior surface of the body of pubis.
- The origin of *pyramidalis* is just above the origin of adductor longus.
- Note the attachments of *gracilis, adductor brevis* and *obturator externus* on the anterior surface of body (from medial to lateral). These attachment also extend further downwards on the outer surface of the conjoined ischiopubic ramus.
- The *obturator internus* arises from the pelvic surface of the body and superior and inferior ramus of the pubic bone.
- The pelvic (posterior) surface of body gives origin to the anterior fibers of *levator ani*.

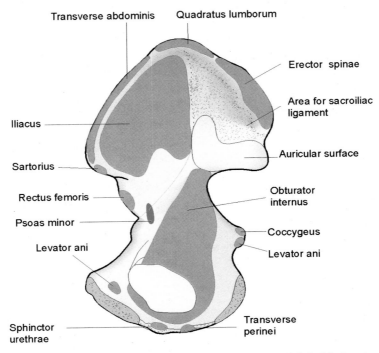

Fig. 3.8: Attachment of muscles on inner aspect of right hip bone

- The *pectineus* arises from the pectineal surface of the superior ramus of pubis.
- *Rectus abdominis* arises from the pubic crest.

ISCHIUM

Muscles Attached to Ischium

- Note the origin of *superior* and *inferior gemelli* in relation to lesser sciatic notch (Fig. 3.7).
- The *quadratus femoris* muscle arises from the femoral surface of the ischium.
- The *obturator externus* arises from the body and ramus of ischium close to the obturator foramen.
- Posterior most fibers of *levator ani* and *coccygeus* muscles arise from the pelvic surface of the ischial spine.
- The origin of muscles from the *ischial tuberosity* is shown in Fig. 3.9. The *adductor magnus* arises from the lower lateral part of ischial tuberosity. The origin also extends on the outer surface of ramus of ischium.
- The *semi-membranosus* arises from the upper lateral part of the ischial tuberosity.

- The upper medial part of ischial tuberosity gives origin to long head of *biceps femoris* and *semitendinosus*.

Attachment of Ligaments and Fascia on the Hip Bone

- The *inguinal ligament* is attached medially on the pubic tubercle and laterally on the anterior superior iliac spine (Fig. 3.10).
- The *conjoined tendon* is attached to the pubic crest and pectin pubis.
- The *lacunar ligament* is attached to the pubic tubercle and pectin pubis.
- The anterior wall of the *rectus sheath* is attached to the pubic crest.
- The *fascia lata* is attached to the outer lip of iliac crest, pubic crest and lower border of the conjoined ischiopubic ramus.
- The anterior and middle layer of *thoracolumbar fascia* is attached to the iliac crest, anterior and posterior to the attachment of quadratus lumborum muscle (Fig. 3.6).
- The superior and inferior fascia of urogenital diaphragm are attached to the conjoined ischiopubic rami.
- The acetabular labrum is attached to the margin of the acetabulum.

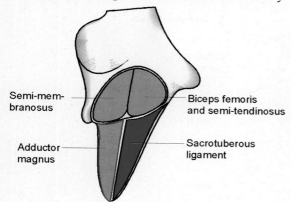

Semi-membranosus

Adductor magnus

Biceps femoris and semi-tendinosus

Sacrotuberous ligament

Fig. 3.9: The origin of muscles from ischial tuberosity

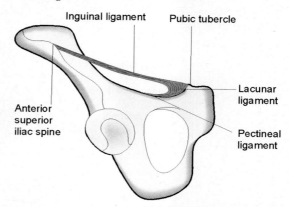

Inguinal ligament

Pubic tubercle

Anterior superior iliac spine

Lacunar ligament

Pectineal ligament

Fig. 3.10: The attachment of inguinal ligament, pectineal ligament and lacunar ligament

- The iliac tuberosity (on the sacropelvic surface) gives attachment to the dorsal and interosseous *sacroiliac ligament*.
- The posterosuperior and posteroinferior iliac spines and posterior border of ilium gives attachment to upper end of the *sacrotuberous ligament*. The lower end of this ligament is attached to the medial margin of ischial tuberosity.
- The *sacrospinous ligament* is attached to the ischial spine (Fig. 3.11).

Blood Vessels and Nerves in Relation to the Hip Bone

- The *pudendal nerve*, nerve to the *obturator internus* and *internal pudendal* vessels lie in relation to the posterior surface of ischial spine (Fig. 3.11).
- The *obturator vessels* and nerve lie close to inferior border of the superior ramus of pubis (in the obturator canal).
- The superior *gluteal vessels* and nerve are in relation to the gluteal surface of ilium (Fig. 3.11).
- Femoral surface of body of ischium is in relation to the *sciatic nerve* and nerve to the quadratus femoris.

Ossification

Hip bone ossifies by three primary centers (Fig. 3.12).

Many secondary centers appear at puberty and fuse with the rest of bone between 20 and 25 years of age (two secondary centers for iliac crest, two for acetabular cartilage, one for anterior inferior iliac spine, one for pubic tubercle and one for pubic crest).

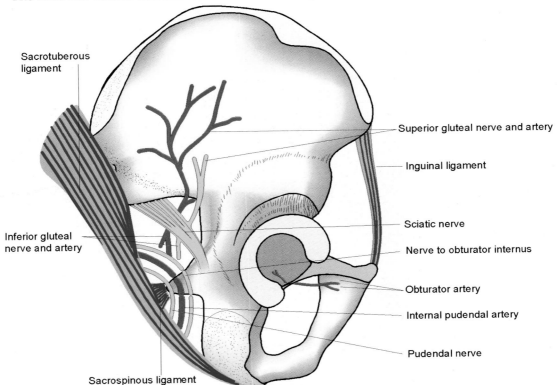

Sacrotuberous ligament

Superior gluteal nerve and artery

Inguinal ligament

Sciatic nerve

Inferior gluteal nerve and artery

Nerve to obturator internus

Obturator artery

Internal pudendal artery

Pudendal nerve

Sacrospinous ligament

Fig. 3.11: Attachment of sacrotuberous and sacrospinous ligaments. Note the relation of blood vessels and nerves

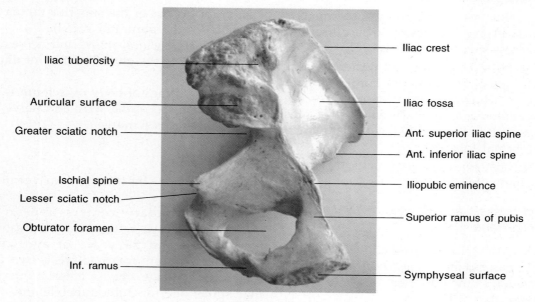

Iliac tuberosity

Auricular surface

Greater sciatic notch

Ischial spine

Lesser sciatic notch

Obturator foramen

Inf. ramus

Iliac crest

Iliac fossa

Ant. superior iliac spine

Ant. inferior iliac spine

Iliopubic eminence

Superior ramus of pubis

Symphyseal surface

Fig. 3A: Inner (pelvic) surface of left hip bone

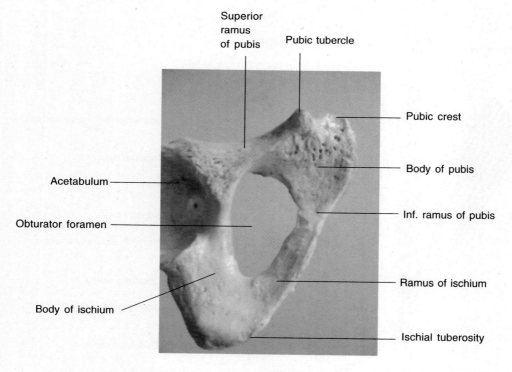

Superior ramus of pubis

Pubic tubercle

Acetabulum

Obturator foramen

Body of ischium

Pubic crest

Body of pubis

Inf. ramus of pubis

Ramus of ischium

Ischial tuberosity

Fig. 3B: External surface of pubis and ischium of right hip bone

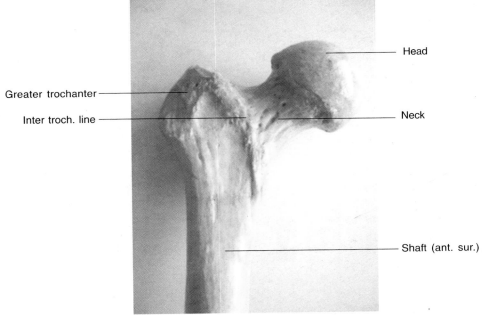

Fig. 3C: Anterior aspect of upper end of right femur

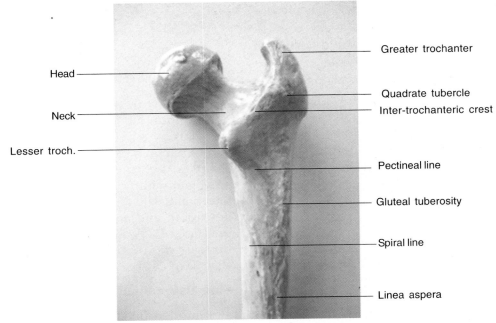

Fig. 3D: Posterior aspect of upper end of right femur

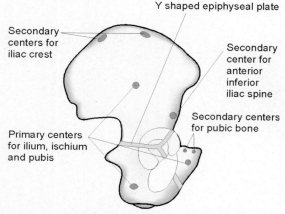

Fig. 3.12: Ossification of hip bone

CLINICAL IMPORTANCE

Fractures

Fractures of hip bone are not very common. They may occur due to roadside accidents or due to sports injuries. The direct anteroposterior compression of hip bone leads to fracture of pubic rami. Lateral compression may produce fracture of the acetabulum. Similarly, a fall on the feet from a roof may lead to fracture of superior margin of the acetabulum.

During sports, a sudden pull of muscles attached on anterior superior and inferior iliac spines, ischial tuberosity and ischiopubic rami may lead to tearing of these bony projections. These kinds of fractures are called as *avulsion fractures*. In this kind of fractures, a small part of bone with a piece of tendon or ligament attached, is torn away.

FEMUR

Femur is the bone of thigh region. It is longest, strongest and heaviest bone in the body. The femur consists of a shaft, an upper end and a lower end (Fig. 3.13). The upper end presents a rounded head, which

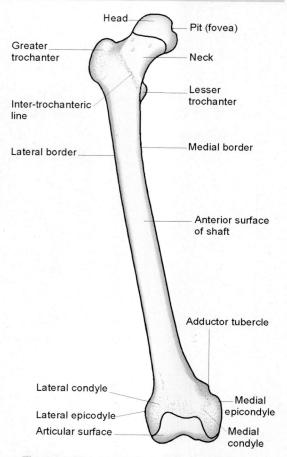

Fig. 3.13: The anterior aspects of right femur

articulates with the acetabulum of the hip bone to form hip joint. The head is joined to the shaft by an elongated neck. The lower end of femur is expanded and presents two *condyles,* i.e., medial and lateral, which articulate with tibia and patella to form the knee joint. The anterior surface of the shaft is smooth and convex forwards. There is presence of a rough and thick vertical ridge (*linea aspera*) on the posterior aspect of the shaft (Fig. 3.14).

Side Determination

* Rounded head is the upper end of the bone.

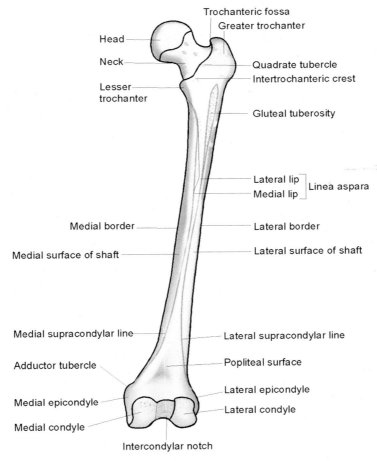

Trochanteric fossa
Greater trochanter
Head
Neck
Quadrate tubercle
Intertrochanteric crest
Lesser trochanter
Gluteal tuberosity
Lateral lip
Medial lip
Linea aspara
Medial border
Lateral border
Medial surface of shaft
Lateral surface of shaft
Medial supracondylar line
Lateral supracondylar line
Adductor tubercle
Popliteal surface
Lateral epicondyle
Medial epicondyle
Lateral condyle
Medial condyle
Intercondylar notch

Fig. 3.14: The posterior aspects of right femur

- Head should be directed upwards, medially and slightly forwards.
- The smooth convex surface of shaft should direct forwards.

Anatomical Position

The shaft of the femur is obliquely placed (lower end of femur is directed downwards and medially). Because the upper ends of two femora are widely separated by two hip bones but two knee joints are placed close to each other when person stands in the anatomical position. As the female pelvis is broader the knee joints are more closely placed in females as compared to males.

- Keep the bone in such a way that head faces upwards, medially and slightly forwards.
- The long axis of shaft should be directed downwards and medially so that the two lower surfaces of both the femoral condyles lie in the same horizontal plane (Fig. 3.15).

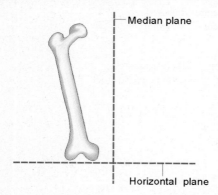

Fig. 3.15: The anatomical position of femur

General Features

The Upper End

The proximal end of the femur consists of a rounded head, neck and two trochanters (greater and lesser).

Head

The head is like a ball, which forms about 2/3rd of a sphere. Near its middle there is the presence of a pit for attachment of *ligamentum teres.*

Neck

The neck connects the head to the shaft. The head and neck makes an angle of about 126 degree with the long axis of body of the femur. Neck has a superior and an inferior border and an anterior and a posterior surface.

Trochanters

Greater and lesser trochanters are two large elevations at the junction of neck with the shaft. The greater trochanter is large, laterally placed quadrilateral mass. This trochanter presents three surfaces (anterior, medial and lateral) and a superior and a

posterior border. The medial surface of greater trochanter presents a deep depression called as *trochanteric fossa.* The lateral surface presents an oblique ridge which runs forwards and downwards.

The lesser trochanter is a conical projection, directed medially and situated on the posteromedial surface at the neck-shaft junction (Fig. 3.16).

Intertrochanteric Line and Crest

The site where the neck joins the shaft, on the anterior aspect, is indicated by the presence of an *intertrochanteric line.* This rough line runs between greater and lesser trochanters. On the posterior aspect, a similar but smoother ridge joins two trochanters. This is known as *intertrochanteric crest*, which marks the junction of neck with the shaft posteriorly. The middle of intertrochanteric crest presents a *quadrate tubercle* (Fig. 3.16).

The Shaft

The shaft or body of the femur shows a slight bowing anteriorly. The shaft is narrowest in the middle but expanded towards upper and lower ends.

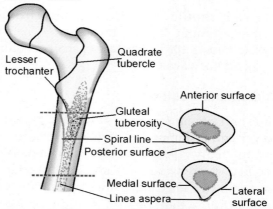

Fig. 3.16: Upper end of femur showing lesser trochanter spiral line and linea aspera

- The shaft presents three surfaces (anterior, medial and lateral) separated by three borders (medial, lateral and posterior).
- The medial and lateral borders are rounded and featureless.
- The posterior border or *linea aspera* is a broad, rough vertical ridge.
- As the linea aspera is broad in the middle part of shaft it presents a medial lip, a lateral lip and an intermediate area.
- When the linea aspera is traced upwards its lateral lip continues as broad rough gluteal tuberosity and the medial lip continues as a narrow rough *spiral line*. The upper end of gluteal tuberosity extends upto the greater trochanter.
- There lies a small triangular surface (posterior surface) between the *gluteal tuberosity* and spiral line in the upper 1/3rd of the shaft (Fig. 3.16).
- When the linea aspera is traced downwards its medial lip continues below as *medial supracondylar line*. Similarly, the lateral lip of linea aspera continues below as *lateral supra condylar line*. The triangular surface between these two lines is called as *popliteal surface*.

Lower End

The lower expanded end of the femur consists of medial and lateral *condyles, intercondylar fossa* and articular surfaces (tibial and patellar) for articulation with tibia and patella.

Two condyles are joined together anteriorly but separated posteriorly by the intercondylar fossa or notch (Figs. 3.13 and 3.14).
- Both the condyles of femur articulate with the corresponding condyles of tibia and patella to form knee joint.

- Each condyle presents five surfaces, i.e., anterior, posterior, medial, lateral and inferior.
- The anterior surfaces of two condyles present an articular patellar surface. It articulates with the posterior surface of patella (Fig. 3.13).
- The outer surface of both the condyles (medial surface of medial condyle and lateral surface of lateral condyle) is rough and convex. The prominent bony point on the outer surfaces of both the condyles are called as *epicondyles* (Fig. 3.17).
- An adductor tubercle is present postero-superior to the medial epicondyle at the lower end of the medial *supracondylar ridge*.
- The inner surface of both the condyles, i.e., lateral surface of medial condyle and medial surface of lateral condyle form the medial and lateral walls of the *intercondylar fossa*.
- The inferior and posterior surfaces of both the condyles are articular and articulate with tibia. Anteriorly, the tibial articular surfaces of both the condyles are continuous with the patellar surface (Fig. 3.17).

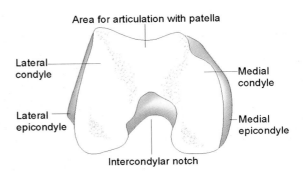

Fig. 3.17: Inferior surface of lower end showing medial and lateral epicondyles and patellar articular surface

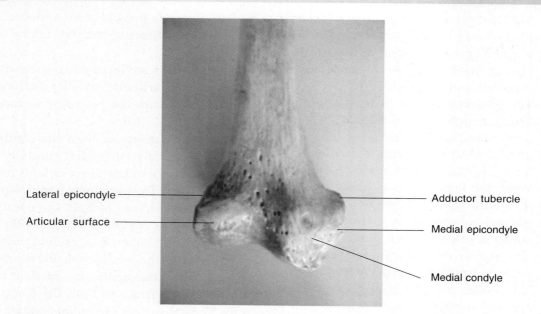

Lateral epicondyle

Articular surface

Adductor tubercle

Medial epicondyle

Medial condyle

Fig. 3E: Anterior aspect of lower end of right femur

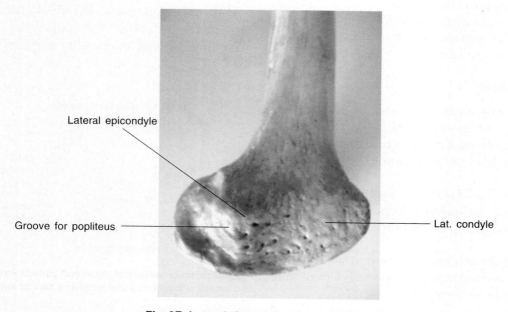

Lateral epicondyle

Groove for popliteus

Lat. condyle

Fig. 3F: Lateral view of lower end of right femur

Particular Features

Muscles Attached on the Upper End of Femur (Figs. 3.18 and 3.19)

- The *obturator internus* and two *gemelli* are inserted on the medial surface of greater trochanter.
- The *obturator externus* is attached into the trochanteric fossa.
- The *piriformis* is inserted on the upper border of greater trochanter.
- The *gluteus minimus* is inserted on the anterior surface of the greater trochanter.
- The *gluteus medius* is inserted on the lateral aspect of greater trochanter.
- The *psoas major* is inserted on the lesser trochanter.
- The *quadratus femoris* is attached on quadrate tubercle.

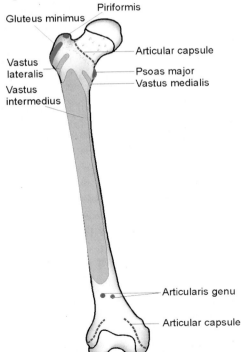

Fig. 3.18: Anterior aspect of right femur showing attachment of muscles

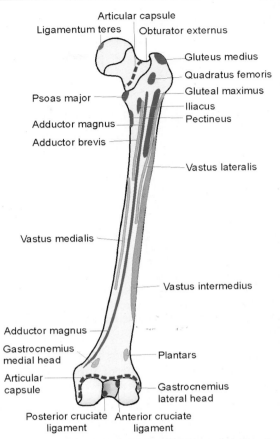

Fig. 3.19: Posterior aspect of right femur showing attachment of muscles. Adductor not shown in this diagram (refer Fig. 3.20)

Muscles Attached on the Shaft of the Femur

- The *iliacus* and *pectineus* are inserted just below the lesser trochanter. The insertion of pectineus lies between gluteal tuberosity and the spiral line.
- A part of the *gluteus maximus* is inserted on the gluteal tuberosity.
- The *vastus medialis* has a linear origin, i.e., from lower part of intertrochanteric line, spiral line, medial lip of linea aspera and upper 2/3rd of medial supracondylar line.
- Similarly, the origin of *vastus lateralis* is also linear. It arises from the upper part of

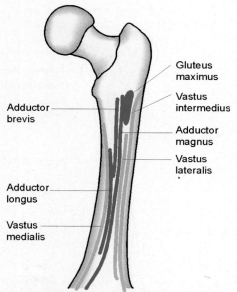

Adductor brevis

Adductor longus

Vastus medialis

Gluteus maximus

Vastus intermedius

Adductor magnus

Vastus lateralis

Fig. 3.20: Attachment of muscles on linea aspera. Attachments of intermuscular septum are not shown here

intertrochanteric line, greater trochan-ter, lateral margin of gluteal tuberosity and lateral lip of linea aspera.

- The *vastus intermediate* originates from the anterior and lateral surface of the shaft.
- Students should note the attachments of the following structures on the linea aspera, from medial to lateral side, with the help of Fig. 3.20. The vastus medialis on medial lip, medial intermuscular septum, adductor brevis (above) and adductor longus (below), adductor magnus, posterior intermuscular septum, short head of biceps femoris, lateral intermuscular septum and vastus lateralis.

Muscles Attached on the Lower End of Femur

- The *popliteus* muscle takes origin from the groove present below the lateral epicondyle.
- The medial head of the *gastrocnemius* arises from the popliteal surface above the medial epicondyle.

- The lateral head of the gastrocnemius arises from the lateral surface of lateral condyle.
- The lower part of the lateral supracondylar line give origin to the *plantaris*.
- The *adductor magnus* is inserted on the medial supracondylar line.
- The tendon of the ischial part of adductor magnus is attached on the adductor tubercle.

Attachments of Ligaments and Intermuscular Septa on the Femur

Few important ligaments and septa are described below:

- The pit or fovea on the head of the femur gives attachment to the *ligamentum teres*.
- *Medial intermuscular septum* is attached on the medial lip of linea aspera and lateral septum is attached on the lateral lip.
- The *posterior intermuscular septum* is attached on the intermediate area of linea aspera.
- The *posterior cruciate ligament* is attached on the lateral surface of the medial condyle (Fig. 3.19).
- The *anterior cruciate ligament* is attached to the medial surface of the lateral condyle (Fig. 3.19).

Blood Vessels in Relation to the Bone

- *Femoral artery* lies anterior to the head of the femur (Fig. 3.21).
- *Popliteal artery* lies on the popliteal surface of the bone.
- Any major nerve is not directly related to femur.

Ossification

The femur ossifies by one primary and four secondary centers (three for upper end and one for lower end (Fig. 3.22).

The lower end is the growing end of the femur.

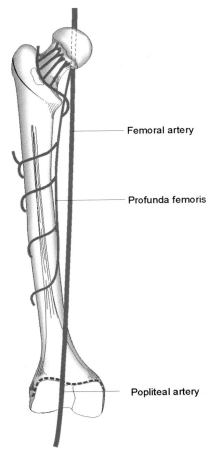

- Femoral artery
- Profunda femoris
- Popliteal artery

Fig. 3.21: Relation of arteries on the posterior aspect of femur

CLINICAL IMPORTANCE

- The secondary center for lower end appears just before birth (ninth months of intrauterine life). The presence of this center indicates that fetus is mature (*viable*) enough to survive after birth. The above fact is used as medicolegal evidence in case if a newborn infant found dead was capable of living at birth or not.

- The fracture of neck of femur is common in old people, especially in females.

- The fracture through the neck of femur is also associated with the injury to blood vessels lying on the surface of neck. These vessels are responsible for the blood supply of the head. Rupture of these blood vessels lead to degeneration of femoral head (*avascular necrosis of head*).

- Fracture of femur between greater and lesser trochanter is also common in old persons.

- Fracture of shaft is usually due to direct injury as in vehicle accidents.

- If the angle of inclination (angle between long axis of body and long axis of neck) is reduced then the condition is called as *coxa vera*. And if this angle is increased the condition is called as *coxa valga* (Fig. 3.23).The normal angle is about 125.

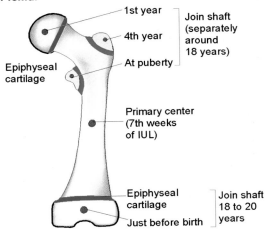

- 1st year
- 4th year — Join shaft (separately around 18 years)
- At puberty
- Epiphyseal cartilage
- Primary center (7th weeks of IUL)
- Epiphyseal cartilage — Join shaft 18 to 20 years
- Just before birth

Fig. 3.22: Ossification of femur

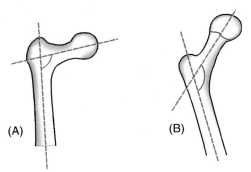

(A)   (B)

Fig. 3.23: (A) Coxa vera and (B) Coxa valga

TIBIA

The skeleton of leg is formed by two long bones, i.e., tibia and fibula. The tibia is the medial weight bearing bone of the leg (Fig. 3.1). It consists of an *upper end* and a *lower end* and a *shaft* or *body* (Figs. 3.24 and 3.25). The upper end of the tibia is expanded and bears medial and lateral condyles. These condyles articulate with the lower end of femur to form knee joint. The lower end of tibia on its medial aspect bears a downward projection called as *medial malleolus*. The shaft or the body of the bone bears a prominent sharp ridge known as *anterior border*. The upper end of anterior border bears a projection called as *tibial tuberosity*.

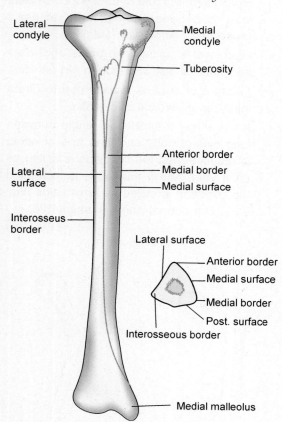

Fig. 3.24: Anterior aspect of right tibia

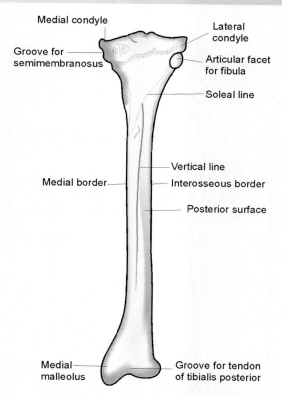

Fig. 3.25: Posterior aspect of right tibia

Side Determination

- The expanded upper end (bearing medial and lateral condyles) should be directed upwards.
- The sharp and prominent anterior border and the tibial tuberosity should be placed anteriorly.
- Medial malleolus at the lower end should face medially.

Anatomical Position

Bone should be kept vertically by holding it in the same hand, to the side it belongs.

General Features

Upper End

The upper end consists of medial and lateral

condyles, an intercondylar area and a tibial tuberosity.

- The upper surface of the medial and lateral condyles is articular in nature. The articular surface of medial condyle is oval and large while that of lateral condyle is small and circular (Fig. 3.26).
- A non-articular rough area is placed between two articular surfaces. This is known as *intercondylar area.*
- There is presence of an elevation in the middle of intercondylar area (intercondylar eminence). This eminence is formed by two tubercles, i.e., medial and lateral *intercondylar tubercles.*
- The posterior surface of medial condyle is deeply grooved.
- The posterolateral surface of lateral condyle bears a circular articular facet for the head of fibula. This articulation is known as *superior tibio-fibular joint.*
- The anterior surface of both the condyles bear a triangular area. The apex of this triangle is directed downwards and there lies a rough projection called as *tibial tuberosity.*

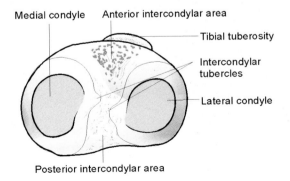

Fig. 3.26: Superior surface of medial and lateral condyles of right tibia

Shaft

The shaft of the tibia is triangular in cross-section, hence presents three borders (anterior, medial and lateral or interosseous) and three surfaces (medial, lateral and posterior).

- The anterior border extends from tibial tuberosity to the anterior margin of medial malleolus. It is sharp, subcutaneous border (Fig. 3.24).
- The *medial border* extends from the medial condyle to the posterior border of the medial malleolus.
- The *lateral* or *interosseous border* extends from lateral condyle to the anterior border of fibular notch at the lower end of tibia.
- The *lateral surface* lies between anterior and interosseous borders.
- The *medial surface* lies between anterior and medial borders. This surface is smooth because it is subcutaneous.
- The *posterior surface* lies between medial and lateral borders. This surface is marked by presence of an oblique soleal line (Fig. 3.25). Thus posterior surface presents a triangular area above soleal line and a medial and a lateral area below soleal line.

Lower End

This end of tibia is much less expanded as compared to upper end. This end projects downwards and medially as the *medial malleolus.* The posterior surface of the malleolus presents a groove. The lateral surface of lower end shows a triangular area (fibular notch) for articulation with the fibula to form inferior tibiofibular joint. The inferior surface of lower end including medial malleolus is articular and articulates with the body of talus to form ankle joint.

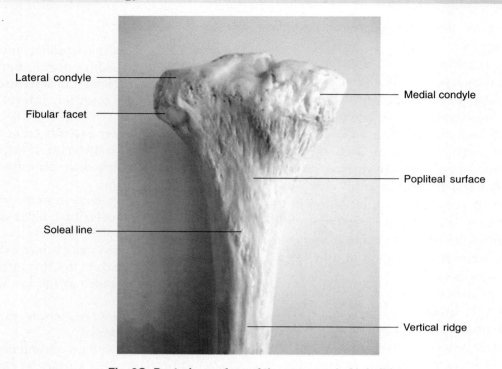

Lateral condyle

Fibular facet

Medial condyle

Popliteal surface

Soleal line

Vertical ridge

Fig. 3G: Posterior surface of the upper end of left tibia

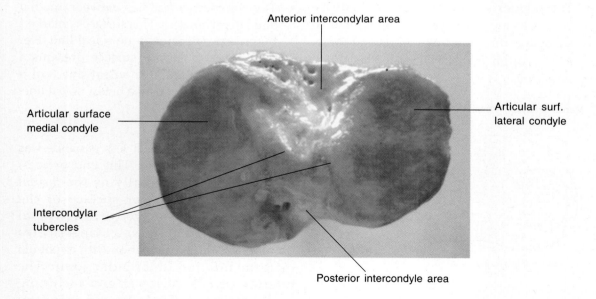

Anterior intercondylar area

Articular surface
medial condyle

Articular surf.
lateral condyle

Intercondylar
tubercles

Posterior intercondyle area

Fig. 3H: Superior surface of condyle of right tibia

Particular Features

Attachment of Muscles on Tibia (Figs. 3.27 and 3.28)

- The tibial tuberosity gives attachment to the *ligamentum patellae* (tendon of quadriceps femoris).
- The *semi-membranosus* is inserted in the horizontal groove on the posterior surface of medial condyle.
- The upper part of media surface receives insertion of three muscles from before backwards, i.e., *sartorius, gracilis* and *semitendinosus*.
- The upper 2/3rd of the lateral surface gives origin to the *tibialis anterior*.
- On the posterior surface of bone, *popliteus* is inserted above the soleal line.

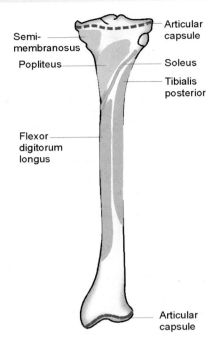

Fig. 3.28: Attachment of muscles on posterior aspect of right tibia

- The soleal line itself gives origin to the *soleus* muscle.
- The medial area below the soleal line, on the posterior surface, gives origin to the *flexor digitorum longus*. While the lateral area gives origin to the *tibialis posterior*.

Attachment of Ligaments on the Tibia

- The anterior and posterior parts of intercondylar area gives attachment to the following structures from before backwards: anterior horn of *medial meniscus, anterior cruciate ligament*, anterior horn of *lateral meniscus*, posterior horn of lateral meniscus, posterior horn of medial meniscus and *posterior cruciate ligament* (Fig. 3.29).
- The lower end of *ilio-tibial tract* is attached on a small triangular area on the anterior surface of the lateral condyle (Fig. 3.30).

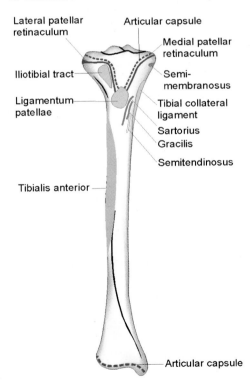

Fig. 3.27: Attachment of muscle on anterior aspect of tibia

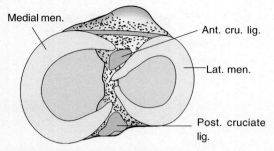

Fig. 3.29: Attachment on the superior surface of medial and lateral condyles of right tibia

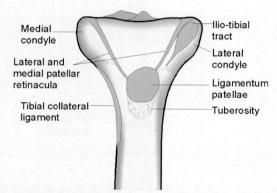

Fig. 3.30: Structures attached on the anterior aspect of the upper end of tibia

- The *tibial collateral ligament* is attached on the medial surface near the upper end of medial border.
- The interosseous or lateral border gives attachment to *interosseous membrane*.
- The fibular notch gives attachment to the *interosseous tibiofibular ligament*.

Tendons, Blood Vessels and Nerves Related to Tibia

- Following tendons, vessels and nerve are related on the anterior aspect of the lower end (from medial to lateral): tibialis anterior, extensor hallucis longus, anterior tibial vessels, deep peroneal nerve, extensor digitorum longus and peroneus tertius (Fig. 3.31).

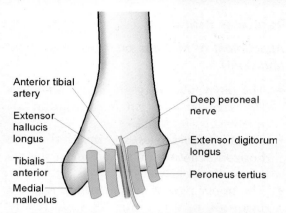

Fig. 3.31: Anterior aspect of lower end of left tibia showing relations of tendons, vessels and nerve

- Following tendons, vessels and nerve are related to the posterior aspect of the lower end of tibia (from medial to lateral side): tibialis posterior, flexor digitorum longus, posterior tibial vessels, posterior tibial nerve and flexor hallucis longus (Fig. 3.32).

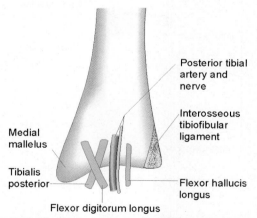

Fig. 3.32: Posterior aspect of lower end showing relation of tendons and vessel

Ossification

Tibia ossifies from three centers, i.e., one primary center for shaft and two secondary centers one each for upper and lower end (Fig. 3.33). Upper end is growing end of tibia.

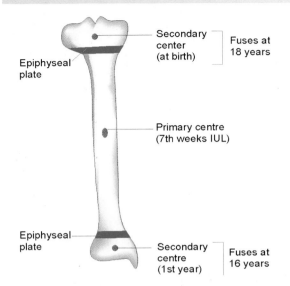

Fig. 3.33: The ossification of tibia

CLINICAL IMPORTANCE

- Most common site for the fracture of tibia is at the junction of middle and lower 1/3rd. This is because tibia is narrowest at this point.
- The fracture of lower 1/3rd of tibia is difficult to heal as this part of tibia is devoid of muscle attachment and periosteal blood supply is poor.
- Tibia is subjected to sever torsion during various sports, which may lead to diagonal fracture of tibial body.
- The body of tibia is also the most common site for compound fracture. In a compound fracture, blood vessels and skin are torn by the fractured end of tibia. This is because tibia is subcutaneous hence skin is easily torn.

FIBULA

The fibula is the lateral bone of the leg. Though the slender fibula has no weight bearing function, but gives attachment to muscles and its lower end (lateral malleolus) takes part in the formation of ankle joint.

The fibula has an upper end, a lower end and an intervening shaft (Figs. 3.34 and 3.35). The upper rounded end is also known as head. The head bears a styloid process and an oval articular surface for articulation with the lateral condyle of tibia. The lower end of fibula is expanded anteroposteriorly to form the *lateral malleolus*. The medial surface of lower end presents a triangular articular surface in front and a depression, the *malleolar fossa*, just posteroinferior to the triangular articular surface.

Side Determination

Side of the fibula can be determined just by looking at its lower end

- Keep the lower end (lateral malleolus) downwards.

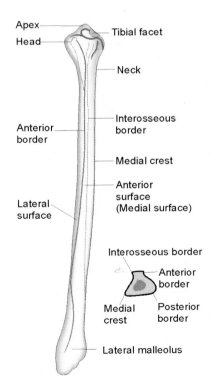

Fig. 3.34: General features of right fibula as seen from front

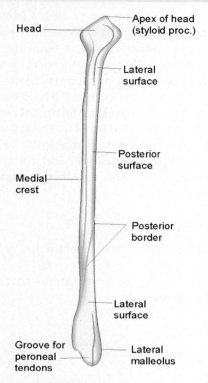

Fig. 3.35: Right fibula as seen from behind

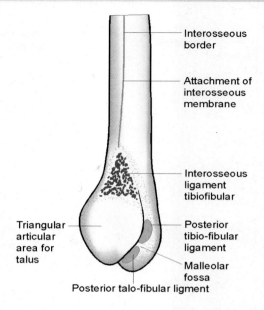

Fig. 3.36: Medial surface at the lower end of fibula

- The triangular articular surface of lateral malleolus should face medially (Fig. 3.36).
- The malleolar fossa should face downwards, backwards and medially.

Anatomical Position

Once you have determined the side of the bone then hold the bone vertically in the hand of same side to which it belongs.

General Features
(Refer Figs. 3.34 and 3.35)

Upper End or Head

- It has a pointed apex known as *styloid process.*
- The superior surface of upper end bears an oval articular facet.
- The neck is the constricted part of the bone just below the head.

Lower End or Lateral Malleolus

- The lateral malleolus presents lateral, medial and posterior surfaces and an anterior border.
- The lateral surface is convex, triangular and continuous above with anterior border. It is subcutaneous surface.
- The medial surface bears a triangular articular facet for the articulation with the talus (Fig. 3.36).
- Behind the facet there is rough depression called as *malleolar fossa.*
- The posterior surface present a groove for tendon.

Shaft

The shaft of the fibula has three borders (anterior, interosseous and posterior) and three surfaces (medial, lateral and posterior).

(As the borders and surfaces of fibula are difficult to identify, take the help of your teacher. Hold the bone in the anatomical position and trace these borders as described below).

Anterior Border

It begins just below the anterior surface of head. Trace this sharp border downwards, near lower end of the bone this border splits to enclose a subcutaneous triangular surface on the lateral aspect of the lateral malleolus.

Interosseous Border

- This border is very close and medial to the anterior border.
- It begins just below the anterior surface of head. When traced downwards it passes medially to end in a rough triangular surface on the medial surface of lower end (Fig. 3.36).

Posterior Border

It extends from the posterior aspect of head to the lateral lip of a groove on the posterior aspect of the lateral malleolus.

Medial (Extensor) Surface

It is a very narrow surface and lies between anterior and interosseous borders. It is also known as anterior surface.

Lateral (Peroneal) Surface

It lies between anterior and posterior borders. At the lower end this surface becomes continuous with the posterior aspect of lateral malleolus.

Posterior (Flexor) Surface

It lies between interosseous and the posterior border. This surface in its upper 2/3rd is divided into medial and lateral parts by a sharp vertical ridge called as *medial crest*.

Particular Features (Refer Figs. 3.37 and 3.38)

Attachment of Intermuscular Septum

- The anterior and posterior borders give attachment to anterior and posterior *intermuscular septum*.
- The interosseous border gives attachment to the *interosseous membrane*.
- The medial crest gives attachment to transverse intermuscular septum.

Attachment of Muscles on Fibula

- The *medial* or extensor surface gives origin to three muscles, i.e., *extensor digitorum*

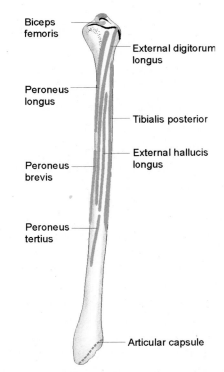

Biceps femoris

External digitorum longus

Peroneus longus

Tibialis posterior

External hallucis longus

Peroneus brevis

Peroneus tertius

Articular capsule

Fig. 3.37: Attachment of muscles on anterior aspect of fibula

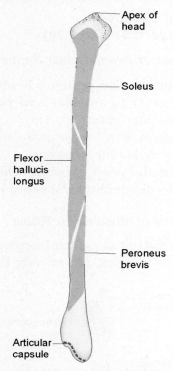

Fig. 3.38: Attachment of muscles on posterior aspect of fibula

longus (from its upper 3/4th surface), *extensor hallucis longus* (from its middle 2/4th) and *peroneus tertius* from lower 1/4th below the origin of *extensor digitorum longus*.

- The *posterior surface* gives origin to *tibialis posterior* from the anterior concave surface lying anterior to the medial crest. The surface posterior to the medial crest gives origin to the *soleus* in upper 3/4th and *flexor hallucis* longus from its lower 3/4th.
- The *lateral surface* gives origin to the *peroneus longus* from its upper 3/4th and *peroneus brevis* from its lower 2/3rd. In the middle third of this surface peroneus brevis lies in front of peroneus longus.
- Lower end of fibula is devoid of muscular attachments.

Tendons and Nerves in Relation to Fibula

- The tendon of peroneus longus and brevis are related to the posterior surface of lateral malleolus (Fig. 3.39).
- The common peroneal nerve is related to lateral aspect of the neck of fibula.

Ossification

The fibula ossifies by three centers. One primary center for shaft and two secondary centers , one each for upper and lower ends (Fig. 3.40).

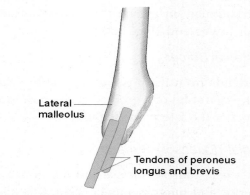

Fig. 3.39: Posterior surface at the lower end of fibula

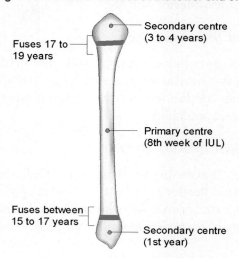

Fig. 3.40: Ossification of fibula

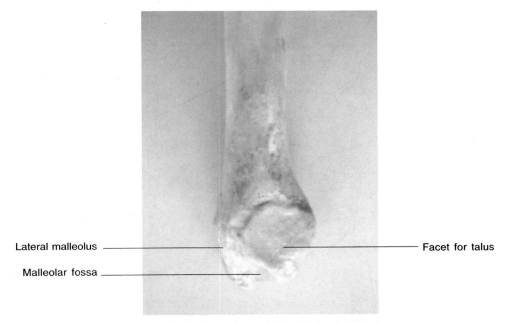

Lateral malleolus

Malleolar fossa

Facet for talus

Fig. 3I: Medial aspect of lower end of left fibula

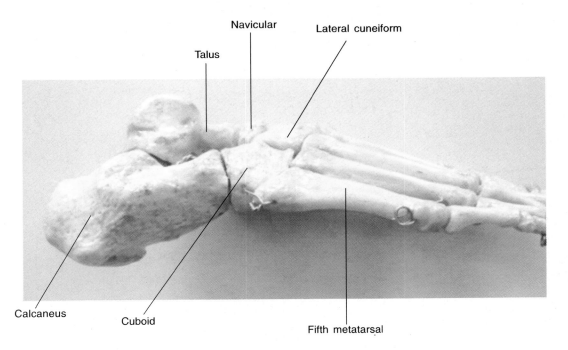

Navicular

Lateral cuneiform

Talus

Calcaneus

Cuboid

Fifth metatarsal

Fig. 3J: Lateral aspect of the articulated right foot

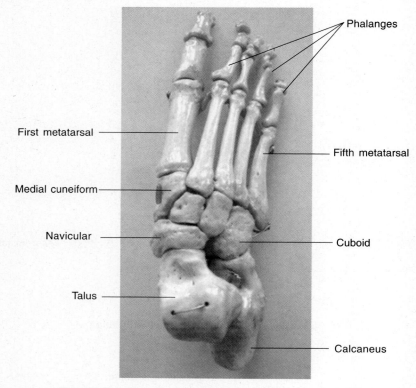

Phalanges

First metatarsal

Fifth metatarsal

Medial cuneiform

Navicular

Cuboid

Talus

Calcaneus

Fig. 3K: Superior (dorsal) aspect of the right articulated foot

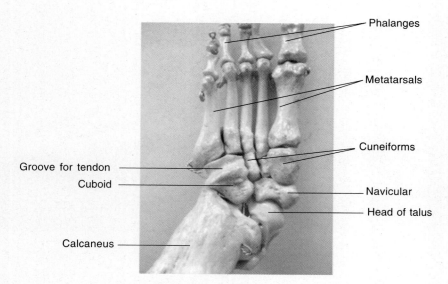

Phalanges

Metatarsals

Cuneiforms

Groove for tendon

Cuboid

Navicular

Head of talus

Calcaneus

Fig. 3L: Plantar aspect of the right articulated foot

Fibula is an exception to the law of *"growing end"* (i.e., the secondary center, which appears first is also the first to fuse with the bone formed by primary center).

CLINICAL IMPORTANCE

- The fractures of fibula commonly occur just above lateral malleolus. These types of fractures are usually associated with the dislocation of ankle.
- Fibula is the bone of choice for bone grafting. The bone grafting is needed when a part of any bone is destroyed by injury, disease or cancer of bone.
- Fibula is chosen for bone grafting because it is non-weight bearing bone. Even if a long piece of this bone is removed, walking, running and jumping is not affected. For the graft, middle third of the bone is used as it has nutrient artery. The piece of bone used for grafting should have periosteum and endosteum intact.

BONES OF THE FOOT

The bones of the foot consists of tarsus, metatarsus and phalanges. Each foot consists of 7 tarsal, 5 metatarsal and 14 phalanges, which are arranged proximodistally. Though we shall study the features of individual bones of foot but students are advised to study an articulated skeleton of foot (Figs. 3.41 to 3.44) to see the arrangement of these bones in relation to each other. In my opinion, the undergraduate students, need not study each and every bone of the foot in detail. Therefore, only two tarsal bones (calcaneus and talus) are described in details.

Tarsal Bones

These are short bones, which form the posterior half of the foot. They are arranged

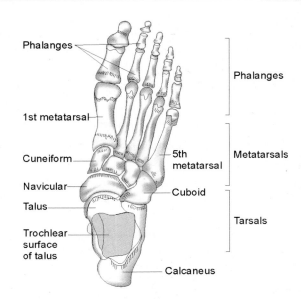

Fig. 3.41: Skeleton of foot as seen from dorsal aspect

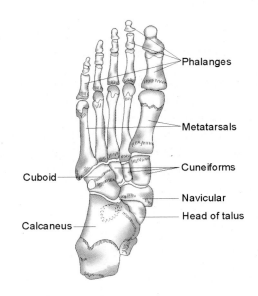

Fig. 3.42: Skeleton of foot as seen from plantar aspect

in three rows. Proximal row consist of talus and calcaneus. The calcaneus is the largest tarsal bone and forms the heel of the foot. Placed above the anterior 2/3rd of calcaneus

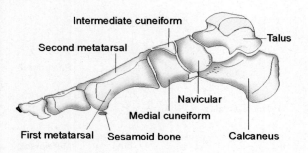

Fig. 3.43: Skeleton of foot as seen from medial aspect

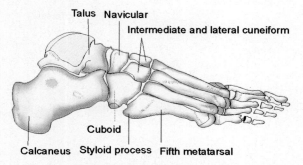

Fig. 3.44: Skeleton of foot as seen from lateral aspect

is another tarsal bone called as talus (Fig. 3.45). The talus articulates with the lower end of the tibia and fibula to form the ankle joint. Anterior to the calcaneus and talus, the middle row is formed by navicular and cuboid bones (Fig. 3.41). The proximal end

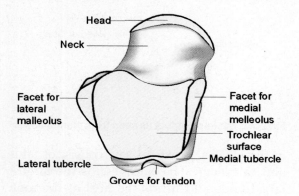

Fig. 3.45: The dorsal surface of talus

of the navicular bone articulates with the head of the talus and is placed medially. The cuboid bone is placed laterally and articulates proximally with calcaneus. The distal surface of navicular bone articulates with other three tarsal bones, i.e., medial, intermediate and lateral cuneiforms (Fig. 3.41).

TALUS

The talus has a *body, neck* and *head*. It is situated on the calcaneus.

Body

- The *superior surface of the body* is articular in nature and bears a large trochlear articular surface for articulation with the lower end of tibia (Fig. 3.45).
- The *medial surface of the body* show a comma shaped articular facet for articulation with the medial malleolus. While lateral surface bears a large triangular facet for articulation with lateral malleolus of fibula.
- The *inferior surface of the body* of the talus presents a concave facet, which articulates with the convex facet on the upper surface of middle third of calcaneus to form *sub-talar joint*.
- The *posterior surface* is narrow and has a groove for a tendon. This groove has a prominent lateral tubercle and a less prominent medial tubercle.

Neck

The neck of the talus projects forwards and medially from the body of the talus. It is non-articular and bears a groove (*sulcus tali*) on its inferior surface (Fig. 3.46).

Head

The rounded head is directed forwards, medially and slightly downwards. Head

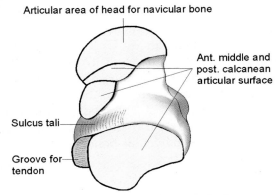

Fig. 3.46: The plantar surface of talus

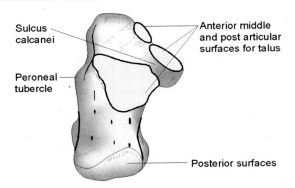

Fig. 3.47: The dorsal surface of calcaneous

bears an extensive convex articular surface, which articulates anteriorly with the navicular bone and below with the upper surface of sustentaculum tali of calcaneus and spring ligament.

The talus is the only tarsal bone that has no muscular or tendinous attachments. The *sulcus tali* gives attachment to the *interosseous talocalcanean* ligament.

Side Determination

- The rounded articular head should be directed forwards.
- The large trochlear articular surface should face upward.
- The large triangular articular surface placed on the side of the body should face laterally.

Anatomical Position

Hold the bone in such a way that head is directed forwards, medially and slightly downwards.

CALCANEUS

The calcaneus is the largest and strongest tarsal bone of the foot (Figs. 3.47 and 3.48). It forms heel and is located below the talus.

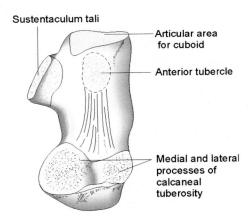

Fig. 3.48: The plantar surface of calcaneous

It articulates superiorly with the talus and anteriorly with the cuboid bone. The calcaneus has six surfaces.

- The *anterior surface* is articular and saddle in shape. It articulates with the cuboid bone.
- The *posterior surface* is non-articular and rough in its middle part for the attachment of tendocalcaneus.
- The medial surface is concave and bears a shelf like projection called sustentaculum tali (Fig. 3.43).
- The *lateral surface* of calcaneus is flat and bears a peroneal tubercle.

- The *plantar* or *inferior surface* of the calcaneus is rough and shows a large prominence on its posterior part called as calcaneal tuberosity. The calcaneal tuberosity presents medial and lateral tubercles. The anterior part of plantar surface bears an anterior tubercle.
- The *dorsal or superior surface* is partly articular and partly non-articular. It bears three articular facets (anterior, middle and posterior facets) for articulation with the corresponding facets on the inferior surface of talus. There is presence of deep groove between middle and posterior facets, *sulcus calcanei*. The sulcus calcanei and sulcus tarsi, in an articulated foot, form *sinus tarsi*.

Side Determination

- The anterior articular surface should face anteriorly.
- The superior surface bearing three articular facets should face upward.
- The sustentaculum tali projects medially.

Anatomical Position

Hold the bone in such a way that the articular area for cuboid should face forwards and laterally with a slight upward inclination.

NAVICULAR

The navicular bone is boat shaped. It articulates distally with the head of talus and proximally with three cuneiforms (Fig. 3.41). The medial surface of the bone bears a navicular tuberosity.

CUBOID

It is the lateral bone extending in the distal row of the tarsus (Figs. 3.41 and 3.42). It is approximately cubical in shape. Proximally it articulates with calcaneus and distally with 4th and 5th metatarsals. On the lateral and inferior aspect it bears a groove for the tendon of peroneus longus. On this aspect, behind the groove, there is the presence of tuberosity (Fig. 3.42). The medial surface of cuboid has articular facets for lateral cuneiform and navicular bone.

CUNEIFORM BONES

These are called as medial, intermediate and lateral cuneiforms. These bones articulate with the navicular proximally and with the bases of 1st, 2nd and 3rd metatarsals distally (Fig. 3.41).

All these bones articulate with each other. The lateral surface of lateral cuneiform also articulates with the cuboid.

THE METATARSAL BONES

The metatarsals are classified as miniature long bones. The five metatarsal bones are numbered from medial to lateral side, i.e., 1st, 2nd etc. The first metatarsal is shortest and strongest as compared to the others. The second metatarsal is the longest (Figs. 3.41 and 3.42). Each metatarsal has a proximally placed base, distally placed head and intervening body (Fig. 3.49). The heads of metatarsals are rounded and articulate with the proximal phalanges. The base of each metatarsal is large as compared to its head and presents five surfaces (medial, lateral, dorsal, plantar and proximal). The base of 5th metatarsal has a large tuberosity for the insertion of the tendon of peroneus brevis.

PHALANGES

Similar to the metatarsals, phalanges are also classified as miniature long bones. The first

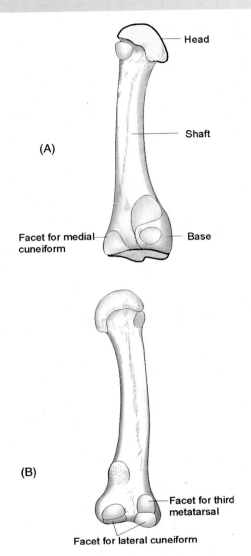

(A)

Head

Shaft

Facet for medial cuneiform

Base

(B)

Facet for third metatarsal

Facet for lateral cuneiform

Fig. 3.49: The second matatarsal of left side (A) medial aspect, (B) lateral aspect

Table 3.1: Differences between metatarsals and metacarpals	
Metacarpals	*Metatarsals*
1. Heads of metacarpals are generally larger or equal in size as compared to their bases.	1. Heads of metatarsals are quite smaller as compared to their bases.
2. Because of the above reason, when we trace the shaft from base towards head it gradually increases in size.	2. Because of the above reason, when we trace the shaft of metatarsal from its base towards the head it gradually decreases in size.

PARTICULAR FEATURES OF THE BONES OF THE FOOT

Insertion of Leg Muscles on the Dorsal Aspect of the Bones of the Foot (Fig. 3.50)

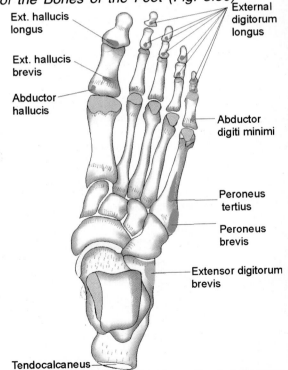

Ext. hallucis longus

External digitorum longus

Ext. hallucis brevis

Abductor hallucis

Abductor digiti minimi

Peroneus tertius

Peroneus brevis

Extensor digitorum brevis

Tendocalcaneus

Fig. 3.50: Insertion of leg muscles on the dorsal aspect of right foot

toe has two phalanges (proximal and distal). The lateral four toes have three phalanges each, i.e., proximal, middle and distal (Fig. 3.41). Each phalanx consists of a proximally placed base, distally placed head and an intervening body. The first toe consists of two phalanges and has only one inter-phalangeal joint. While, rest of the toes have proximal and distal interphalangeal joints.

- The *peroneus brevis* is inserted on the lateral aspect of the base of fifth metatarsal bone.
- The *peroneus tertius* is attached on the dorsal aspect of the base of fifth metatarsal.
- The *extensor digitorum longus* is attached on the base of middle and distal phalanges of lateral four toes.
- The *extensor hallucis longus* is inserted on the base of distal phalanx of great toe.
- The *tendocalcaneous* is inserted on the middle of the posterior surface of the calcaneous.

Attachment of Muscles on the Plantar Aspect of the Bones of Foot (Fig. 3.51)

- The *flexor hallucis longus* is inserted into the base of distal phalanx of the great toe.
- The *flexor digitorum longus* is inserted into the plantar surface of the bases of the distal phalanges of lateral four digits.

- The *peroneus longus* muscle is inserted on the base of first metatarsal and on the lateral aspect of the medial cuneiform bone.
- The *tibialis anterior* is inserted into the medial cuneiform and base of first
- metatarsal on the medial and plantar aspects.
- The *tendon of tibialis posterior* has very extensive insertion. It is mainly inserted into the tuberosity of the navicular bone and medial cuneiform. This tendon also sends slips to all other tarsal bones (except talus) and bases of 2nd, 3rd and 4th metatarsals.

Origin and Insertion of the Intrinsic Muscles of the Foot

The dorsal aspect gives origin to the *extensor digitorum brevis* (Fig. 3.50). On the plantar surface many intrinsic muscles are attached

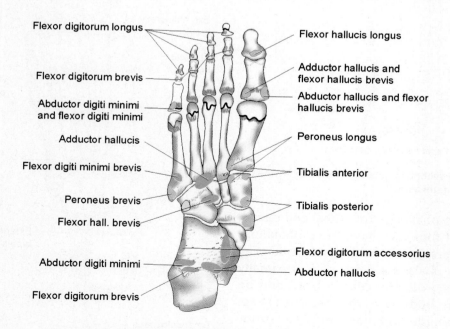

Flexor digitorum longus

Flexor digitorum brevis

Abductor digiti minimi and flexor digiti minimi

Adductor hallucis

Flexor digiti minimi brevis

Peroneus brevis

Flexor hall. brevis

Abductor digiti minimi

Flexor digitorum brevis

Flexor hallucis longus

Adductor hallucis and flexor hallucis brevis

Abductor hallucis and flexor hallucis brevis

Peroneus longus

Tibialis anterior

Tibialis posterior

Flexor digitorum accessorius

Abductor hallucis

Fig. 3.51: Attachment of muscles on plantar aspect of right foot

(flexor digitorum brevis, abductor digiti minimi, abductor hallucis, flexor digitorum accessorius, flexor hallucis brevis, adductor hallucis and flexor digiti minimi brevis). Students should learn the origin and insertion of all these muscles with the help of Fig. 3.51. The origin and insertion of *plantar interossei* is shown in Fig. 3.52 and that of *dorsal interossei* in Fig. 3.53.

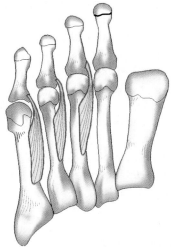

Fig. 3.52: Origin and insertion of plantar interossei

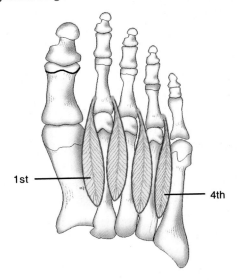

1st

4th

Fig. 3.53: Origin and insertion of dorsal interossei

Attachment of Ligaments on the Bones of the Foot (Fig. 3.54)

The bones of the foot give attachment to many ligaments. Few important ligaments are described here:

- The *interosseous talocalcaneal ligament* is attached between sulcus tali of talus and sulcus calcanei of calcaneus.
- The *spring ligament (plantar calcaneonavicular ligament)* is attached on the anterior margin of sustentaculum tali of the calcaneus and to the plantar surface of the navicular bone.
- On the plantar surface the *long plantar ligament* is attached posteriorly on the tuberosity of the calcaneus and anteriorly to the cuboid bone and bases of 2nd, 3rd and 4th metatarsal bones.

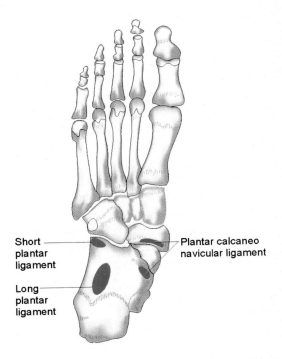

Short plantar ligament

Plantar calcaneo navicular ligament

Long plantar ligament

Fig. 3.54A: Attachment of ligaments on the plantar aspect of foot

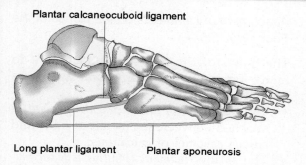

Plantar calcaneocuboid ligament

Long plantar ligament   Plantar aponeurosis

Fig. 3.54B: Attachment of ligaments on the plantar aspect of foot, as seen from lateral aspect

- The *short plantar ligament* is proximally attached to the anterior tubercle of calcaneus and distally on the cuboid.
- The groove on the posterior aspect of the talus is related to the tendon of *flexor hallucis longus*.

CLINICAL IMPORTANCE

- A fall from height on the heel may break calcaneus into several pieces.
- The fracture of the neck of talus may occur due to sudden and severe dorsiflexion.
- The fracture of metatarsal may occur due to fall of heavy object on the foot.
- Fatigue fractures of the metatarsals may result from prolonged walking.
- Os trigonum is the name given to an occasional small bone present on posterior aspect of the talus. This results when the bone of lateral tubercle fails to unite with the body of the talus. The presence of os trigonum, in a radiograph, may be mistaken as a fracture.

Ossification

Tarsal Bones

Calcaneus ossifies by one primary center and one secondary center. All other tarsal bones ossify by one center only (Fig. 3.55). The ossification of metatarsal and phalanges are also shown in Fig. 3.55.

PATELLA

The patella is also known as kneecap as it lies in front of the knee joint. It is a small triangular bone present in the tendon of quadriceps femoris. Patella is not a true bone as it is devoid of periosteum, hence it is classified as sesamoid bone.

The patella has an apex, a base, medial and lateral borders, an anterior and a posterior surface (Figs. 5.56 and 3.57). The base forms the upper border of the bone. The apex is directed downwards. The anterior surface is rough and subcutaneous while posterior surface is mostly articular. The articular surface is divided into a smaller medial and a large lateral surface by a vertical ridge (Fig. 5.57). These surfaces articulate with the corresponding surfaces on the femoral condyles.

Side Determination

- The apex of patella should be directed downwards.
- The smooth articular surface should face posteriorly.
- The larger lateral part of the articular area should lie on the lateral side.

The anterior surface is rough (presents number of longitudinal ridges). The base, medial and lateral border give attachments to many muscles (Fig. 3.58). The posterior surface is mostly articular. Only a small portion near the apex is rough and gives attachment to the ligamentum patellae (Fig. 3.58). The articular surface is divided into a large lateral and a small medial articular area by a vertical ridge (Fig. 3.57).

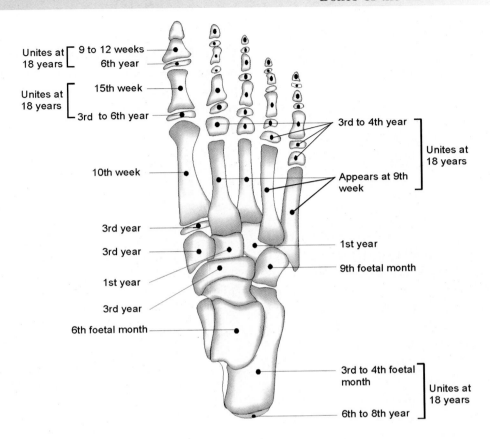

Fig. 3.55: Ossification of bones of foot

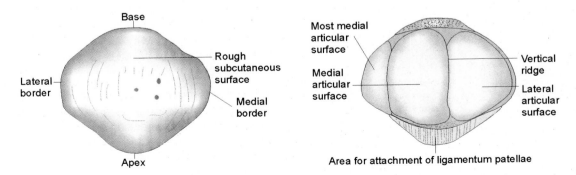

Fig. 3.56: The anterior surface of right patella

Fig. 3.57: The posterior (articular) surface of right patella

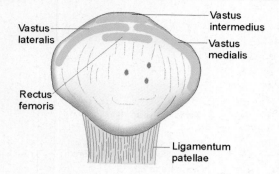

Fig. 3.58: The attachment of patella

These articular surfaces comes in contact with the reciprocal patellar articular surface of femur, i.e., larger lateral area of patella with lateral femoral condyle and medial area with medial condyle. The medial articular area is further separated by a vertical ridge from the most medial narrow strip, which comes in contact with medial condyle of femur during full flexion.

As the patella moves downwards when knee is flexed, its articular areas move on the articular areas at the lower end of femur. The various articular areas coming in contact with the femur (from extension to full flexion) are shown in Fig. 3.59.

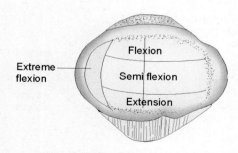

Fig. 3.59: Various articular areas coming in contact with femur during extension and flexion

Ossification

The patella is cartilaginous up to three years of age. Several ossification centers appears in patella between 3 to 6 years of age. These centers unite with each other and complete the ossification.

FURTHER DETAILS

The correlation between articular area of a bone and the magnitude of stress it resists

Pal and Routal (1991) studies the above correlation in various bones. They found that there exist a significant positive correlation between area of the articular surface and magnitude of stress passing through it. This indicates that the area of articular surface increases or decreases as per the increase or decrease in the magnitude of stress it resists. Similarly, they also found a significant positive correlation between development of bone (bone mass) and its articular area. This indicates that bone mass (development) runs parallel to the articular area. Thus this study could reveal that the articular area and bone development are related to the stress acting on bone.

Determination of age from hip bone

By studying the ossification of many short and long bones of the body, age can be determined till the end of second decades. The basisphenoid suture closes at around 25 years of age. The hip bone serves as important tool to determine the age of an adult person (upto 60 years of age).

The medial (symphyseal) surface of pubic bone shows the horizontal ridges and grooves that show changes with increasing age. Todd (1920) was the first to use pubic symphysis for age determination. Mckern and Stewart (1957) revised the criteria of Todd. Pal and Tamankar (1983) undertook a study to find out how far

Todd's and Mckern and Stewart criteria were applicable to Indian pubic bone. They found that Indian specimens showed overage with Todd's criteria and the same specimens showed underage on using Mckern and Stewart criteria.

Determination of sex from hip bone

The hip bone is the most commonly used bone in medicolegal examination of sex of human skeletal remains. A study by Pal *et al.* (2002) observed that many of commonly used parameters were not much reliable. The only parameter which could identify the large number of bones was based on measurements of the greater sciatic notch (Singh and Potturi, 1978). However, this study has some drawbacks. Pal *et al.* (2009) worked out an excellent parameter, i.e., index *"height of pelvic cavity/length of arcuate line"* which identified a large percentage of male and female bones with 100% accuracy.

The trabecular architecture of the tarsal bones

The complexity in the spongy bone of foot has fascinated investigators for about 150 years. In past many investigators from India have studied the trabecular architecture of the tarsal bones (Singh, 1978; Sinha, 1975 and Pal, 1990). Among all the tarsal bones, talus possesses the most difficult architecture to study and

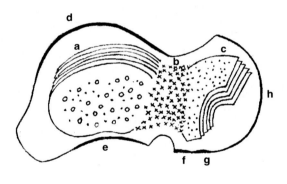

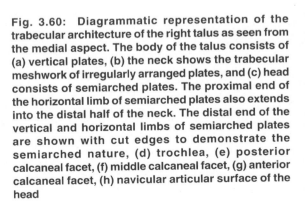

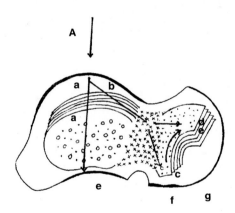

Fig. 3.60: Diagrammatic representation of the trabecular architecture of the right talus as seen from the medial aspect. The body of the talus consists of (a) vertical plates, (b) the neck shows the trabecular meshwork of irregularly arranged plates, and (c) head consists of semiarched plates. The proximal end of the horizontal limb of semiarched plates also extends into the distal half of the neck. The distal end of the vertical and horizontal limbs of semiarched plates are shown with cut edges to demonstrate the semiarched nature, (d) trochlea, (e) posterior calcaneal facet, (f) middle calcaneal facet, (g) anterior calcaneal facet, (h) navicular articular surface of the head

Fig. 3.61: Diagrammatic representation of the force transmission through the talus. During midstance, the vertical compressive force (A) is brought by the tibia on the talus, part of which (a) goes directly downward on the posterior calcaneus facet, and from the anterior ends of vertical plates of the body, (b) the force is also transmitted to the trabecular meshwork of the neck, (c) compressive force acting on the vertical limbs of semiarched plates, (d) tensile force acting ont he horizontal limbs of semiarched plates, (e) at the end of the stance phase, when the heel starts rising and the foot is supinated, the compressive force from the vertical limbs of the semiarched plates is shifted to the horizontal limbs

correlate with function. This is because talus receives the load from tibia and fibula and passes it downwards to calcaneus and forwards to navicular bone. Pal and Routal (1998) studied the architecture of cancellous bone of talus (Fig. 3.60) and correlated with the mechanical stress to which talus is subjected during standing and walking (Fig. 3.61).

Very recently Athavale *et al.* (2010) have studied the trabecular architecture of calcaneus in detail and correlated with its clinical significance.

Further Readings

* Todd T.W. (1920) *Am. J. Phy. Anthropol.* (U.S.A.) 258.
* McKern T.W. and Stewart T.D. (1957) *Technical Report* EP45 (U.S.A.) 71.

* Singh I (1978), *Journal of Anatomy* (U.K.) 127: 305-310.
* Singh S and Potturi BR (1978) *Journal of Anatomy* (U.K.) 125, 619-624.
* Pal G.P. and Tamankar B.P. (1983) *Indian J. Med. Res.* 694-701.
* Sinha D.N. (1985), *Journal of Anatomy* (U.K.) 140: 111-117.
* Pal G.P. (1990) *The J. of ASI* 39, 1-11.
* Pal G.P. and R.V. Routal (1991). *The Anatomical Record* (U.S.A.) 230: 570-574.
* Pal G.P. and Routal R.V. (1998), *The Anatomical Record* (U.S.A.) 252: 185-193.
* Pal G.P., Bose S and Choudhary S.M. (2002) *J. of ASI* 51, 134.
* Pal G.P., Bose S. and Choudhary S.M. (2009) *J. of ASI* 58(2), 173-178.
* Athavale S.A., Joshi S.D. and Joshi S.S. (2010), *Surgical and Radiological Anatomy* 32, 115-122.

4 Bones of the Vertebral Column

The vertebral column is present in the central region of the body. It is the main constituent of the axial skeleton. The column is also called as *spine* or *backbone*. The vertebral column extends from the base of the skull to the tip of the coccyx.

The vertebral column is composed of a series of many irregular bones called as vertebrae (Fig. 4.1). There are 33 vertebrae in the column, which are connected to each other by *intervertebral joints*. The important intervertebral joint is made up of fibrocartilagenous *intervertebral disc* that binds bodies of two adjacent vertebrae. The length of vertebral column is about 70 centimeters in an adult male. About 1/4th length of the column is formed by intervertebral discs. The adult vertebral column is divided into 5 different regions:

- **The Cervical Region:** This part of the column is present in the neck and consists of seven cervical vertebrae.
- **The Thoracic Region:** It is present in thorax and consists of 12 thoracic vertebrae.
- **The Lumbar Region:** It is present in the abdominal part and is made up of 5 lumbar vertebrae.
- **The Sacral Region:** It is present in the pelvic region and consists of five fused sacral vertebrae. These five fused vertebrae are considered as a single bone, the sacrum.
- **The Coccygeal Region:** It is present at the lower end of the column. It is usually a single bone, which is formed by the fusion of four coccygeal vertebrae.

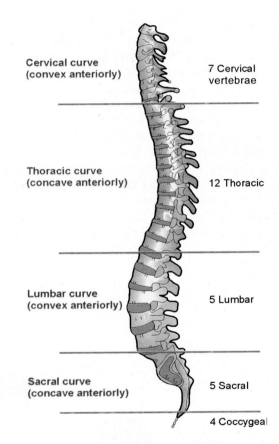

Cervical curve
(convex anteriorly)

7 Cervical
vertebrae

Thoracic curve
(concave anteriorly)

12 Thoracic

Lumbar curve
(convex anteriorly)

5 Lumbar

Sacral curve
(concave anteriorly)

5 Sacral

4 Coccygeal

Fig. 4.1: The vertebral column (spine) as seen from lateral side

When you shall view the articulated vertebral column from front (anterior aspect) you shall notice the progressive increase in the width of the vertebral bodies from above downwards (from C2 to L5). This is due to the fact that at each vertebral segment some more load is added to the column.

Curves of the Vertebral Column

When viewed from the lateral side, the vertebral column of an adult shows four curvatures, i.e., *cervical, thoracic, lumbar and sacral* (Fig. 4.1).

- The cervical and lumbar curves are convex anteriorly, while thoracic and sacral curves are concave anteriorly.
- The thoracic and sacral curvatures are called *primary curvatures*. They are present at the time of birth. These curvatures are formed mainly due to the shapes of vertebrae.
- The cervical and lumbar curvatures are called as *secondary curvatures* because they develop after birth. Cervical curvature develops after the child starts holding the head on the neck. The lumbar curvature develops after an infant assumes upright posture and begins to walk. Thus secondary curvatures develop due to the posture (Fig. 4.2). In adults, cervical and lumbar intervertebral discs are thicker anteriorly thus contributing to anterior convexity. The posterior aspect of the column is formed by laminae, spinous processes and articular facets. The adjacent spinous process and laminae are inter-connected with the help of ligaments, while facets form joints.

Functions of the Vertebral Column

- The vertebral column acts as a rigid but flexible column.
- It transmits the weight of the body.
- It supports the head.
- The vertebral column protects the spinal cord and part of the spinal nerves.
- It gives attachments to the ribs and muscles of the back.

STRUCTURE AND FUNCTIONS OF A TYPICAL VERTEBRA

In the following paragraphs only the

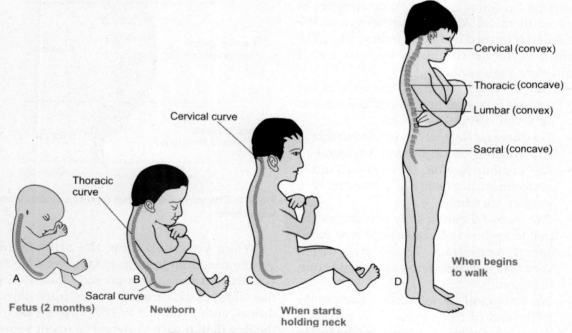

Fig. 4.2: The curvatures of vertebral column

generalized description of vertebrae is given. The detailed description of cervical vertebrae is given in Chapter 7, for thoracic vertebrae in Chapter 5 and for lumbar, sacral and coccyx in Chapter 6.

Though the vertebrae of different regions of the vertebral column vary in size, shape and other characteristics but there are many basic features that are common in these vertebrae. A vertebra from the mid thoracic region is best suited to study the basic features of a typical vertebra. Following description of a typical vertebra is based on the features of a mid thoracic vertebra (Figs. 4.3 and 4.4).

A typical vertebra consists of:
- A vertebral body.
- A vertebral (neural) arch with seven processes.

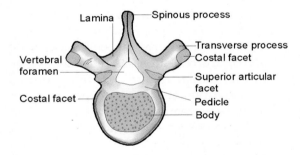

Fig. 4.3: A typical thoracic vertebra as seen from superior aspect

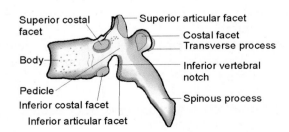

Fig. 4.4: A typical thoracic vertebra as seen from lateral aspect

Vertebral Body

Hold a typical thoracic vertebra in your hand and note the following:
- The body of a vertebra is situated anteriorly. It is somewhat cylindrical in shape.
- The cylindrical body is rounded from side to side. Its superior and inferior surfaces are flat.
- Thus body has six surfaces (anterior, posterior, superior, inferior and two lateral).
- The anterior, lateral and posterior surfaces contain minute foramina for the vessels.
- The body is made up of spongy bone and covered by a thin layer of compact bone. However, its superior and inferior surfaces are not covered by compact bone but by a thin layer of hyaline cartilage in living persons. The upper and lower surfaces give attachments to the intervertebral discs.

Vertebral Arch

The vertebral arch is situated posterior to the body of vertebra. It consists of a pair of pedicles and laminae (Fig. 4.3). Seven processes arise from the vertebral arch of a typical vertebra.

Pedicles

- The pedicles are short, stout bars that are attached on the posterolateral aspects of the body.
- They are attached close to the superior border of the body (Fig. 4.4).
- Pedicles project posteriorly and somewhat laterally from the body to unite with the laminae.
- If we look at the lateral aspect of a vertebra there is presence of *inferior vertebral notch* just below the pedicle. This notch is bounded anteriorly by the body,

superiorly by pedicle and posteriorly by the inferior articular process.

- The *superior vertebral notch* is situated above the pedicle. It is much shallower as compared to the inferior vertebral notch.

Laminae

- These are flat vertical plates of the bone that join in midline to form the posterior portion of the vertebral arch.
- They extend backwards and medially from the pedicles.
- Posteriorly, the lamina of right and left sides fuse with each other in midline to form spinous process (Fig. 4.3).
- The body, pedicles and laminae of a vertebra together enclose a foramen called *vertebral foramen.*
- Collectively the vertebral foramina of the successive vertebrae form the vertebral canal that transmits the spinal cord.

Transverse Processes

- The transverse process extends laterally on each side from the point where lamina and pedicle join each other.

Articular Processes

- There are two superior and two inferior articular processes. They also arise from the junction of pedicle and lamina.
- Each articular process bears a smooth *articular facet.* In the thoracic vertebrae, the superior articular facets face postero-laterally, while inferior ones, face antero-medially.

Spinous Process

- It projects posteroinferiorly in midline from the junction of two laminae (Fig. 4.3).

Functions of the Various Components of a Vertebra

- The bodies and intervertebral discs are involved in the transmission of the load of the trunk to the lower limbs.
- The intervertebral discs are shock absorbers and also permit various movements between two successive bodies.
- Articular processes (and facet joints) allow and guide the movements between adjacent vertebrae.
- Facet joints are also involved in the transmission of load. The magnitude of load transmitted by facet joints varies in various regions of the column, i.e., cervical and lumbar facets are highly loaded while thoracic are least loaded.
- Lamina is also involved in the transmission of load as it is passing from superior to inferior articular facet joints.
- In the thoracic region, where the column is concave anteriorly, the load passes from vertebral arch (lamina) to the body. While, in the lumbar region, where column is concave posteriorly, load passes from body to vertebral arch. The transmission of load between body and vertebral arch is through the pedicles.
- The spinal cord and its meninges are well protected in the vertebral foramen (canal).
- The transverse and spinous processes give attachment to muscles and act as levers for various movements of the vertebral column.
- Transverse processes in the thoracic region are also involved in transmission of load from ribs to the laminae.

Articulation between Two Successive Typical Vertebrae

The articulations between two successive

thoracic vertebrae are shown in (Figs. 4.5A and 4.5B). Adjacent vertebrae are connected to each other at three intervertebral joints, i.e., one median joint between bodies and two joints between the articular processes of successive vertebrae. The two adjacent vertebral bodies are joined by the intervertebral disc, which is made up of fibrocartilage. Each disc consists of *annulus fibrosus* (outer fibrous part) and *nucleus pulposus* (inner soft part).

The two superior articular processes of a vertebra articulate with the two inferior articular processes of the vertebra situated above it. Similarly, two inferior articular processes of the vertebra articulate with the two superior articular processes of the vertebra situated below it. The joints between articular processes are synovial in nature and are also known as *facet joints.*

The vertebral foramina of the successive vertebrae from a continuous vertebral canal, that contains spinal cord and its meninges. The superior and inferior vertebral notches

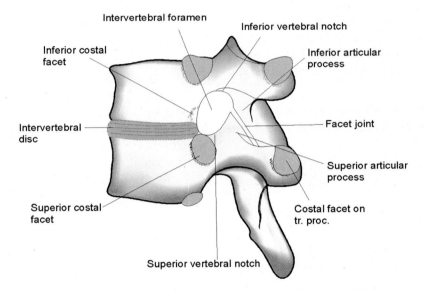

Fig. 4.5 A: Joints between two successive thoracic vertebrae

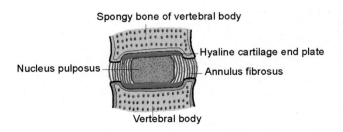

Fig. 4.5 B: The diagrammatic representation to show the structure of intervertebral disc

of the adjacent vertebrae join to form the intervertebral foramen through which passes the spinal nerves and vessels (Figs. 4.6A and 4.6B). The boundaries of intervertebral foramen are formed anteriorly by the body of upper vertebra, intervertebral disc and a small part of the body of lower vertebra. The upper and lower boundaries are formed by pedicles of upper and lower vertebrae respectively. Posterior boundary is formed by the lamina of upper vertebra and facet joint (Fig. 4.5A).

The articular facets are present on the body and transverse processes of the thoracic vertebra. These are called as costal facets. The costal facets of adjacent bodies articulate with the head of the rib. The facet on the transverse process articulates with the tubercle of the rib.

Principle Distinguishing Features of the Vertebrae of the Various Regions of the Vertebral Column

Besides the features mentioned in the Table 4.1, following features will help students to distinguish cervical, thoracic and lumbar vertebrae from one another:

- A cervical vertebra can be easily identified because of the presence of a foramen in its transverse process. This foramen is called as *foramen transversarium* (Fig. 4.7).
- A thoracic vertebra is recognized by the presence of articular facets on the body and transverse processes. These facets are called as *costal facets,* which articulate with the ribs (Fig. 4.3).
- A lumbar vertebra is recognized because it has a large kidney shaped body (Fig. 4.8). There is absence of foramen transversarium in the transverse processes. There is also the absence of costal facets on the body and transverse processes.
- The sacrum is easily identified because of its shape. As it is formed by the fusion of five sacral vertebrae, it is a single, curved and triangular bone (Fig. 4.9).
- The coccyx is formed by the fusion of four coccygeal vertebrae. Coccyx is identified by its small size and fused nature (Fig. 4.9).

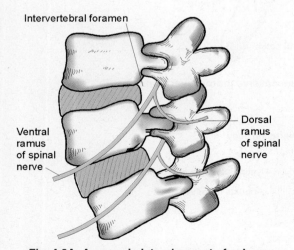

Fig. 4.6A: As seen in lateral aspect of column

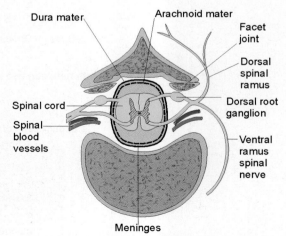

Fig. 4.6B: As seen in the transverse section of column

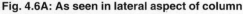

Figs. 4.6A and B: Figures showing structures passing through intervertebral foramen

Table 4.1: Comparison of structural features of typical cervical, thoracic and lumbar vertebrae			
	Cervical	*Thoracic*	*Lumbar*
Overall structure of vertebra	Shown in Fig. 4.7	Shown in Fig. 4.3	Shown in Fig. 4.8
Overall size of vertebra	Small	Larger	Largest
Body	Small and wider from side to side than anteroposteriorly	Heart shaped, has one or two costal facets for the head of rib	Large and kidney shaped
Pedicles	Strong and directed backwards and laterally	Thin flattened from side to side and directed backwards	Thick and directed backwards and laterally
Vertebral foramen	Triangular and large	Circular and small	Triangular and small as compared to the cervical vertebrae
Direction of superior articular facets	Facets directed posterosuperiorly	Facets directed posterolaterally	Facets directed posteromedially
Direction of inferior articular facets	Facets directed anteroinferiorly	Facets directed anteromedially	Facets directed anterolaterally
Transverse processes	Small and bears a small foramen, anterior and posterior tubercles	Long and thick, directed posterolaterally, bears costal facets for tubercle of rib	Long and slender
Foramen transversarium	Present in Tr. Proc.	Absent	Absent
Spine	Short and bifid	Long, pointed and directed posteroinferiorly	Thick, quadrilateral and directed posteriorly

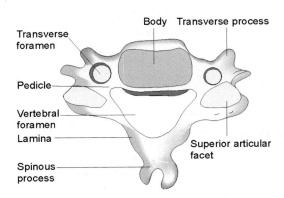

Fig. 4.7: A typical cervical vertebra as seen from superior aspect

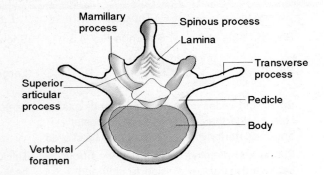

Fig. 4.8: Typical lumbar vertebra as seen from superior aspect

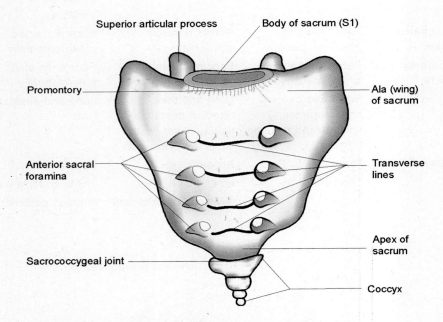

Fig. 4.9: Sacrum and coccyx as seen from anterior aspect

Movements Occurring in the Vertebral Column

As the sacral and coccygeal vertebrae are fused with each other, no movements are possible between these vertebrae. The cervical, thoracic and lumbar vertebrae are not fused hence, are mobile. Two adjacent vertebrae are joined with each other at three intervertebral joints, i.e., by intervertebral disc (between two adjacent bodies) and by two synovial joints (between articular

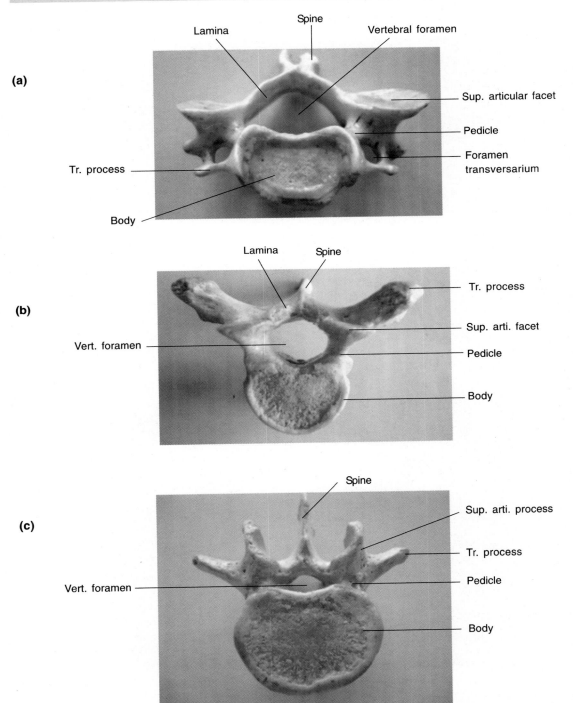

Fig. 4A: (a) Superior aspect of typical cervical, (b) typical thoracic, and (c) a typical lumbar vertebra

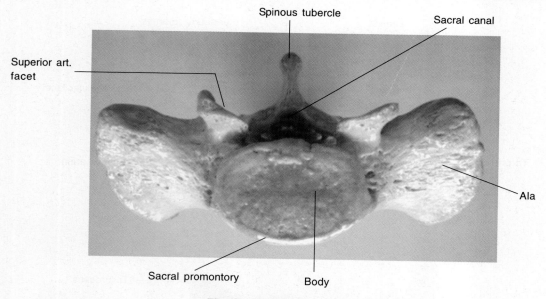

Spinous tubercle

Sacral canal

Superior art. facet

Ala

Sacral promontory

Body

Fig. 4B: Superior view of sacrum

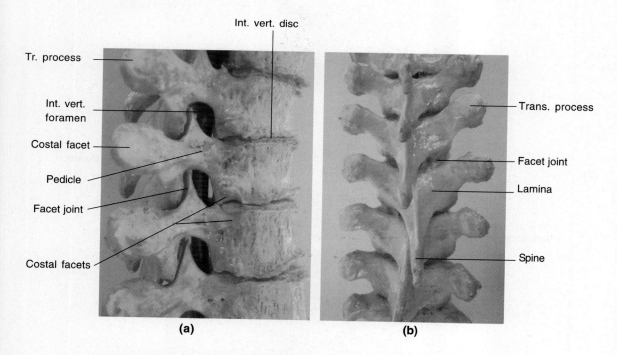

Int. vert. disc

Tr. process

Int. vert. foramen

Costal facet

Pedicle

Facet joint

Costal facets

Trans. process

Facet joint

Lamina

Spine

(a)

(b)

Fig. 4C: (a) Right lateral, and (b) posterior view of articulated thoracic column

processes). The movements between two adjacent vertebrae are slight. But when movements between series of vertebrae are added, the column shows the considerable flexibility.

Following movements are possible in the vertebral column:

- *Flexion*: Forward bending (Fig. 4.10A).
- *Extension*: Backward bending (Fig. 4.10B).
- *Lateral flexion*: Side bending (Fig. 4.10C).
- *Rotation*: Twisting (Fig. 4.10D).

In different regions, i.e., cervical and lumbar regions are more mobile as compared to thoracic. Almost all types of movements are possible in cervical region. Rotation movement is the main movement of thoracic region, but this movement is not possible in lumbar region.

Particular Features of a Typical Vertebra

There are many ligaments, which connect adjoining vertebrae. With the help of these ligaments and intervertebral joints a flexible but rigid column is formed.

Attachments of Ligaments (Fig. 4.11)

- The anterior longitudinal ligament is attached on the anterior surfaces of the

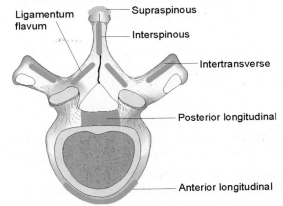

Fig. 4.11: Attachment of various ligaments on a vertebra

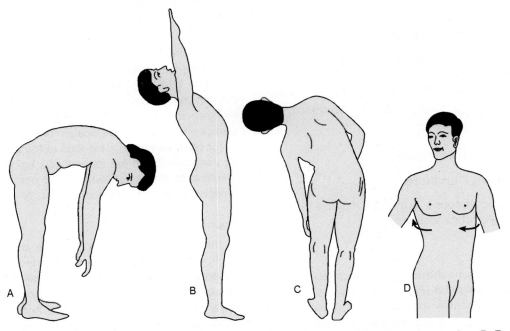

Figs. 4.10A to D: Movements of the vertebral column. A- Flexion, B- Extension, C- Lateral flexion, D- Rotation

bodies of successive vertebrae. It is a continuous ligament, which extends from the base of the skull to the sacrum.

- The posterior longitudinal ligament is also a continuous ligament and attached on the posterior surface of the bodies of vertebrae.
- The transverse processes of the adjacent vertebrae are connected by intertransverse ligaments.
- Ligamentum flava connect the laminae of adjacent vertebrae.
- Similarly, the spinous processes of adjacent vertebrae are connected by interspinous ligaments.
- In the cervical region the tips of spines are connected by the elastic ligament, called as ligamentum nuchae.
- The supraspinous ligaments are attached on the tips of spinous processes of vertebrae between 7th cervical vertebra to the sacrum.

Attachments of Muscles

Various muscles are attached on the various aspects of vertebrae in different vertebral regions. The attachments of these muscles are described along with the bones of that region.

CLINICAL IMPORTANCE

Abnormal Curvatures

Following abnormal curvature may be present in the vertebral column:

Kyphosis

This is due to the abnormal increase in the thoracic curvature (Fig. 4.12A) (increase in the thoracic concavity anteriorly). It is usually seen in old age due to osteoporosis. The osteoporo-

sis leads to the erosion of the anterior part of one or more vertebrae, leading to increase in concavity.

Lordosis

This is due to the abnormal increase in lumbar curvature (Fig. 4.12B) (increase in the lumbar convexity anteriorly). This results due to the weakness of the abdominal muscles. Lordosis may also occur in obese people and pregnant ladies. This is due to the shift in the line of gravity because of increase in the weight of abdominal contents.

Scoliosis

It is the most common deformity of the vertebral column and predominantly observed in girls in the teens. In this condition, there is an abnormal lateral curvature associated with the rotation of the vertebrae (Fig. 4.12C). In most of the cases cause of the scoliosis is not known. Known causes are hemivertebra, maldevelopment of one upper limb, asymmetry in the length of the lower limbs.

Fractures

The fracture of the vertebral column may occur due to forceful flexion or hyperextension of the column. The forceful sudden flexion of the column may occur due to fall from the height on feet or the head. This leads to the compression fracture and dislocation of one or more successive vertebrae. This kind of fracture may be associated with the injury to the spinal cord resulting in loss of sensation and paralysis of muscles below the level of injury.

Spondylolysis

In this condition there occurs the breakage (cleft) in the vertebral arch (at lamina between superior and inferior articular processes) of one or both sides. This condition is common in lower lumbar region (Figs. 4.13A and 4.13B). Spondylolysis may result due to excessive

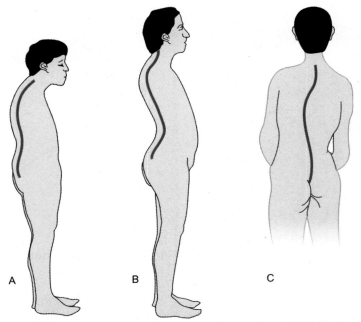

Fig. 4.12A: Kyphosis is an increase in throcic concavity

Fig. 4.12B: Lordosis is an increase in lumbar convexity

Fig. 4.12C: Scoliosis is abnormal lateral curve

mechanical stress. It is now considered as the fatigue fracture of lamina. This condition is different from spondylolisthesis (described below). In spondylolysis there is no displacement of the vertebral body and it is often asymptomatic (without pain).

Sponaylolisthesis

In this condition there occurs breakage in laminae between superior and inferior articular processes. The spondylolisthesis is usually observed at the level of L5 vertebra. In this condition the vertebral body, two pedicles and superior articular processes are displaced anteriorly (Fig. 4.14). While the inferior articular processes, laminae and spinous process retain normal position with the arch of sacrum.

Tuberculosis of the Spine

The vertebral bodies are the common sites for the tubercular infection. This is due to the spongy nature of vertebral body and rich blood supply. Due to the infection, the spongy bone of the body is destroyed and pus is formed. This leads to the collapse of vertebral bodies as the load of trunk is brought by upper vertebrae.

FURTHER DETAILS

New Concepts for the Load Transmission Through Vertebral Column

Though the vertebral column is formed by the vertebral bodies and neural arches, only the bodies are generally considered to be responsible for weight bearing, the neural arches merely contributing to the formation of the verterbral canal. The articular processes are considered to determine the range and direction of movement between any two vertebrae. However, the works of Denis (1983) and Louis (1985) have claimed that facet joints are also involved in weight bearing. Both have put forward the "three column spine" concept for spinal stability. Similarly, Pal and Routal (1986)

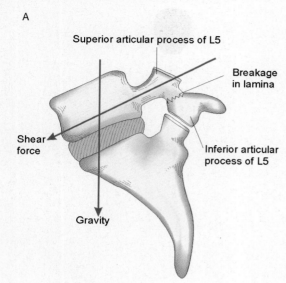

A

Superior articular process of L5

Breakage in lamina

Shear force

Inferior articular process of L5

Gravity

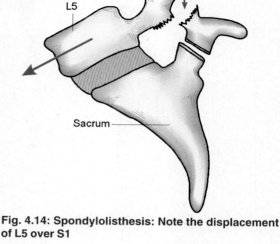

Breakage in the lamina of L5

L5

Sacrum

Fig. 4.14: Spondylolisthesis: Note the displacement of L5 over S1

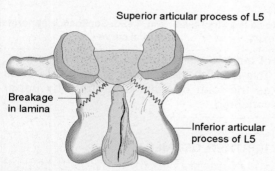

Superior articular process of L5

Breakage in lamina

Inferior articular process of L5

B

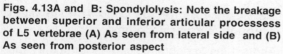

Figs. 4.13A and B: Spondylolysis: Note the breakage between superior and inferior articular processess of L5 vertebrae (A) As seen from lateral side and (B) As seen from posterior aspect

reported that the vertebral column not only transmits weight through bodies and inter-vertebral discs but also through the neural arch. In the cervical part of the vertebral column weight is transmitted through three columns, i.e., an anterior column formed by bodies and intervertebral discs and two posterior columns formed by the articular pillars (Fig. 4.15). However, because of the incorporation of bar-like articular processes into the laminae at the

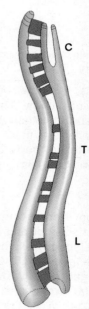

C

T

L

Fig. 4.15: Diagrammatic representation of weight transmission through the various regions of the vertebral column. In the cervical region (C) weight is transmitted through three columns while in the thoracic (T) and lumbar (L) regions it is transmitted through two columns. Thick black staples connecting the two columns represent pedicles. Note the direction and thickness of pedicles. Pedicles are shown on one side only and only few are drawn

level of C7 and below, these two separate posterior columns cannot be traced in the thoracic and lumbar regions (Fig. 4.16). According to Pal and Routal (1987) the load in thoracic and lumbar regions is transmitted through two parallel columns, one anterior (formed by bodies and intervertebral discs) and one posterior (formed by successive articulations of laminae with each other at their articular facets).

Pal (1989) investigated the route and relative magnitude of weight passing through different components of the sacrum (see Chapter 6).

Magnitude of load passing through three columns in cervical region and two columns in thoracolumbar regions

In the cervical region the bodies and intervertebral discs carry about 54% and two posterior columns 46% (23% each) of the total load. In the upper thoracic region, where only two columns are present, around 75% of load is transmitted through anterior column formed by the vertebral bodies. The posterior column formed by laminae carries only about 25% of the total load acting on the vertebral column. However, at T12 segment 85% load passes through body (anterior column) and 15% through lamina. Again at L4 level 81% of load passes through body and 19% through lamina. These findings indicated that there occurs the shifting of load between anterior and posterior columns through pedicles. As the cervical column is concave posteriorly, the two posterior columns are highly loaded. Because of anterior concavity of thoracic column weight is transferred from posterior to anterior column through the anteriorly inclined pedicles. And in the lumbar region, where concavity is posterior, a part of the compressive force of anterior column is transmitted to the posterior. Thus the compressive force in the curvilinear column tends to deviate towards the line of gravity (Fig. 4.17). Pedicles play an important role in this shifing of the load. The shifting of the load between

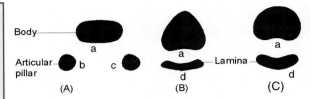

Fig. 4.16: Diagrammatic representation of the of positions of weight bearing pillars of the vertebral column in the (A) cervical, (B) thoracic, and (C) lumbar regions; (a) cross-section of anterior column formed by bodies; (b) and (c) cross-sections of posterior column formed by articular porcesses; (d) cross-section of posterior column formed by lamina

body and neural arch has been confirmed with the help of trabecular bone study (Pal et al., 1988).

The Orientation of the Articular Facets of Facet Joints

The direction of orientation of superior articular facets are different in cervical (Fig. 4.3), thoracic (Fig. 4.7) and lumbar regions (Fig. 4.8). In the mid cervical region they face posteromedially. In thoracic region they are flat and face posterolaterally, while in lumbar region they face posteromedially and become curved. Pal et al. (1999 and 2001) reported that the orientation of the C3 superior articular facets was always posteromedially (Fig. 4.18). The posteromedially facing facets of C3 prevent the rotational movement between C2/C3 joints, thus keeping C2 vertebra in fixed position so that atlas can move side to side along with head, at atlantoaxial joint. At C5, facets face coronally but at C6 they face posterolaterally. Thus the cervical superior facets change their direction from posteromedial to posterolateral mostly at C5/C6 joint. This kind of orientation facilitates rotational movements.

Pal and Routal (1999) investigated the possible mechanism for the change in orientation, i.e., from a posterolaterally facing superior articular facet in thoracic region to a posteromedially

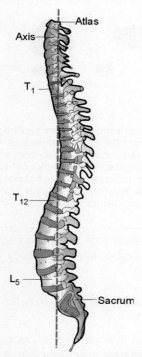

Fig. 4.17: Line of gravity (vertical pecked line) in relation to the vertebral column curvature

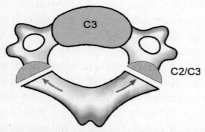

Fig. 4.18: Figure showing the C2/C3 facet joints where both the superior articular facets face posteromedially. The superior articular facets of C3 prevent the rotational movement between C2/C3 joints, thus keeping the C2 vertebra in a fixed position

facing curved articular surface in the lumbar region. Most of the column showed a gradual change extending over 2 to 3 successive vertebrae. The study suggested that the change in the orientation of the superior articular process, from posterolateral to posteromedial

plane occurred due to change in the direction of weight transmission through facet joints at thoracolumbar junction. In thoracic region posterolaterally facing facets helped in transmission of load from posterior to anterior column (from lamina to body through facet joint and pedicle (Fig. 4.19). This is in accordance with the passage of line of gravity (Fig. 4.17). In lumbar region as the line of gravity passes posterior to column the posteromedially facing superior articular facets help in the transfer of load from body to lamina through pedicle.

The change in the direction of facets occur gradually at T11 and T12 vertebrae because the line of gravity crosses these two vertebrae while going from anterior to posterior side. Because of gradual rotation of superior facet at T11 and T12 level the posterior margin of superior articular facet comes close to mamillary tubercle which eventually fuses with it (Fig. 4.20).

Thus the characteristic posteromedially facing concave superior articular process of lumbar vertebrae have formed because of the fusion of the articular process and the mamillary tubercle.

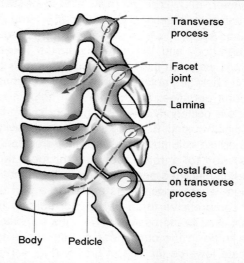

Fig. 4.19: Lateral aspect of a part of thoracic column. Arrows indicate the route of the weight transmission from ribs to the bodies of the lower vertebrae

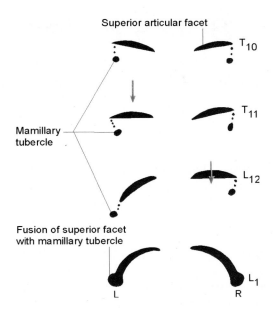

Superior articular facet

T_{10}

Mamillary tubercle

T_{11}

L_{12}

Fusion of superior facet with mamillary tubercle

L_1

L   R

Fig. 4.20: Diagrammatic representation of a column showing gradual change in the orientation of superior articular processes between thoracic 10 (T10) and lumbar first (L1) vertebrae. The gradual rotation of the superior articular process brings it close to mamillary tubercle, which ultimately fuses with it. Thus the posterior most part of lumbar articular process is formed by the fused mamillary tubercles which, morphologically, is an integral part of the transverse process

Further Readings

- Denis F. (1983). *Spine* (Am. vol.) 8, 817-824.
- Louis R. (1985). *Anatomia Clinica* 7, 33-42.
- Pal G.P. and Routal R.V. (1986). *Journal of Anatomy* (U.K.) 148, 245-261.
- Pal G.P. and Routal R.V. (1987). *Journal of Anatomy* (U.K.) 152, 93-105.
- Pal G.P., Leocosio and Routal R.V. (1988). *The Anatomical Record* (New York) 222, 418-425.
- Pal G.P. (1989) *Journal of Anatomy* (U.K.) 162, 9-17.
- Pal G.P. and Routal R.V. (1999), *Journal of Anatomy* (U.K.) 195, 199-209.
- Pal G.P., Routal R.V. and Saggu S.K. (2001), *Journal of Anatomy* (U.K.) 198, 431-441.

5 | *Bones of the Thoracic Region*

The skeleton of the thoracic region forms a bony cage, which protects lungs, heart and some upper abdominal organs. This cage is formed by the following bones and cartilages:

- Thoracic vertebrae and intervertebral discs.
- Ribs and costal cartilages.
- The sternum.

The thoracic cage is narrower at its superior end and broader at its inferior end.

The cage is flattened anteroposteriorly. Posteriorly, it is formed by 12 thoracic vertebrae and intervertebral discs. The sidewalls of this cage are made up of 12 ribs on each side (Fig. 5.1A). The posterior end of each arched rib articulates with the vertebral column. The anterior end of each rib is attached to the costal cartilage. Through these costal cartilages, ribs gain attachment to the sternum (Fig. 5.1B). The sternum is a

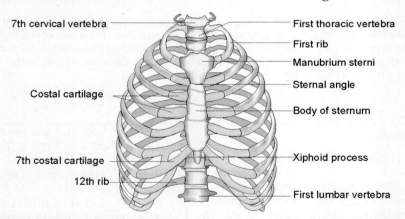

Fig. 5.1A: The thoracic cage as seen from anterior aspect. The thoracic cage is formed, posteriorly, by 12 thoracic vertebrae

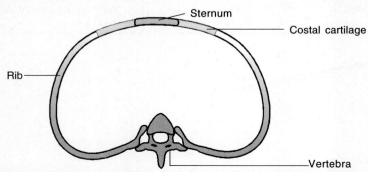

Fig. 5.1B: Vertebra, ribs, costal cartilages and sternum forming the thoracic cage

flat narrow bone situated on the anterior aspect of the thoracic cage.

STERNUM

The sternum is a flat, elongated bone measuring about 6 inches in length. It is situated anteriorly in the wall of the thorax. From above downwards sternum consists of three portions, i.e., the *manubrium, the body* and the *xiphoid process* (Fig. 5.2). The body is the middle and largest portion of the sternum. The junction of the manubrium and the upper end of the body forms the *manubriosternal joint* (the *sternal angle*). The junction of the lower end of the body and xiphoid process forms *xiphisternal joint*.

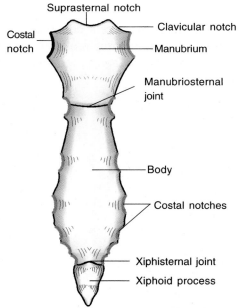

Fig. 5.2: Parts of sternum as seen from front

General Features

Manubrium

- The manubrium is the widest and thickest of the three parts of sternum. It is roughly quadrilateral in shape.

- The upper border of the manubrium is concave. It is known as *suprasternal notch*.
- Lateral to the suprasternal notch are *clavicular notches* that articulate with the medial ends of the clavicles to form *sternoclavicular joints*.
- Inferolateral to the clavicular notch there lies a *costal notch* where the first costal cartilage articulates with the manubrium to form *sternocostal joint*. This joint is classified as *synchondrosis* (primary cartilagenous joint).
- The manubrium and the body of the sternum lie in different planes at the *manubriosternal joint*, therefore the joint projects forwards. This projecting angle is called as *angle of Louis* or *sternal angle* (Fig. 5.3).

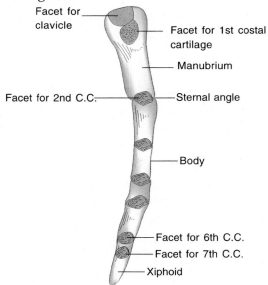

Fig. 5.3: The lateral view of sternum

- At the sternal angle, the second costal cartilage articulates with the lower end of the manubrium and the upper end of the body.
- As the sternal angle is projecting and subcutaneous it is an easily palpable

landmark. This fact is utilized to count the ribs. The rib counting starts with the 2nd rib adjacent to the sternal angle.

- The lower end of the manubrium lies at the level of the lower border of T4 vertebra.

Body of the Sternum

The body of the sternum is long and thin plate of bone. Its lateral borders present costal notches for articulation with 2nd to 7th costal cartilages (Fig. 5.3). All these joints are synovial in nature. In the adults the body of sternum is made up of four pieces (*sternebrae*). These pieces of bones are joined to each other by primary cartilagenous joints. These joints begin to fuse soon after puberty. In an adult, these fusion sites are seen as three transverse ridges.

Xiphoid Process

The xiphoid process is the smallest, triangular part of the sternum. The upper end of the xiphoid process meets the body of the sternum to form *xiphisternal joint*. The lateral border of xiphoid process has a demifacet for articulation with 7th costal cartilage.

The xiphoid process is cartilaginous in young people. It begins to ossify at about third year of age. It gets completely ossified at about 40 years of age. It fuses with the body of the sternum in old people.

Particular Features

Attachments of Muscles on Anterior Surface of the Sternum

Note the origin of the sternal head of the *sternocleidomastoid* and *pectoralis major* muscles

and insertion of *rectus abdominis* with the help of Fig. 5.4.

Muscles attached on the posterior aspect of the sternum.

Note the origin of sternohyoid, sternothyroid and sternocostalis with the help of Fig. 5.5. Also note the reflection of pleura on both the sides of sternum.

Ossification

The sternum develops by the fusion of right and left cartilaginous plate in midline. After the fusion many centers of ossification appear in the cartilaginous model (Fig. 5.6).

CLINICAL IMPORTANCE

Fractures

Sternal fractures may occur due to automobile accidents. The sternum is broken into pieces due to crush injuries against steering wheel.

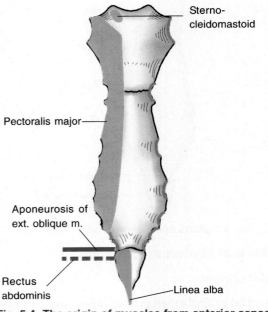

Fig. 5.4: The origin of muscles from anterior aspect of sternum

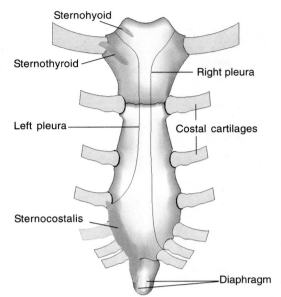

Fig. 5.5: Note the attachment of muscles and relation of pleura on the posterior aspect of sternum

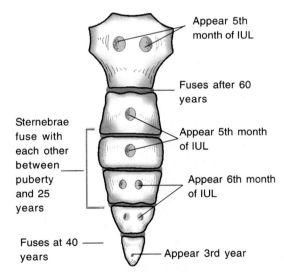

Fig. 5.6: The ossification of sternum

Sternotomy

For coronary bypass surgery and surgeries on lung, these organs are exposed by cutting the sternum in midline. A wide gap is exposed between two splitted parts of sternum because of elasticity of costal cartilages and flexibility of ribs. After surgery two splitted parts of the sternum are joined by wire sutures.

Bone marrow biopsy

As the sternum is superficial (subcutaneous) it is best suited for needle biopsy of bone marrow. The bone marrow sample is obtained from the spongy bone of sternum with the help of needle. The bone marrow biopsy is needed to diagnose blood abnormalities and for bone marrow transplantation.

Sternum is helpful in identification of sex

To a certain extent the sex of individual can be identified with the help of sternum as the female sternum is short and wide as compared to males, Jit, *et al.* (1980). The determination of the sex of bones is needed in medico-legal cases.

Congenital defects of sternum

As the sternum develops by the fusion of two halves of sternum in midline, if these two pieces fail to fuse then the heart is exposed on the thoracic wall (*ectopia cordis*). In this condition pericardium also fails to form.

Sometimes there may be the presence of a foramen in the body of sternum. This occurs due to faulty ossification.

RIBS

Ribs are curved, flat bones that form the greater part of the thoracic wall. They are arranged in twelve pairs. The length of the ribs increases from the first to seventh rib. Thereafter the length gradually decreases from eighth to the twelfth rib. Each rib articulates posteriorly with corresponding vertebra. The anterior ends of ribs (except eleventh and twelfth ribs) articulate with the sternum through costal cartilages.

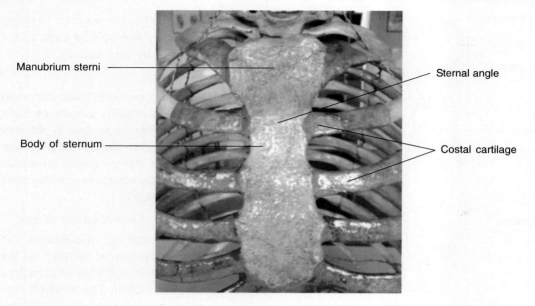

Manubrium sterni

Sternal angle

Body of sternum

Costal cartilage

Fig. 5A: Thoracic cage as seen from anterior aspect

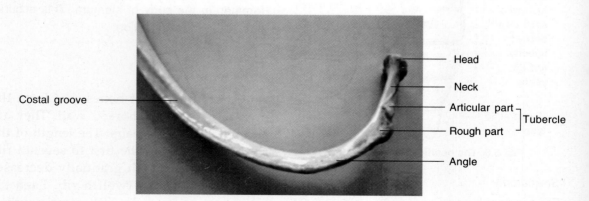

Costal groove

Head

Neck

Articular part ⎤
                ⎬ Tubercle
Rough part ⎦

Angle

Fig. 5B: Inferior aspect of the right typical rib

Classification of Ribs

There are three types of ribs (Fig. 5.7):

True Ribs

These ribs are directly attached to sternum through their own costal cartilages. The first seven ribs are true ribs and these ribs are also called as *vertebrosternal ribs*.

False Ribs

These ribs are indirectly connected to the sternum. Their costal cartilages are joined to the costal cartilages of superior ribs. The eighth to the tenth ribs are false ribs and are also called as *vertebrochondral ribs.*

Floating Ribs

The eleventh and twelfth ribs are not connected with the sternum. Their anterior ends are free and covered by rudimentary costal cartilage. They are also known as *vertebral ribs or floating ribs.*

Ribs may also be classified as *typical* and *atypical ribs.* The typical ribs are those, which have same (common) features. The 3rd to the 9th ribs are typical ribs. The atypical ribs have special features therefore can be differentiated from the rest of the ribs. The atypical ribs are 1st, 2nd, 10th, 11th and 12th ribs.

The Typical Ribs

A typical rib consists of head, neck, tubercle, angle and shaft (Figs. 5.8 and 5.9). The head

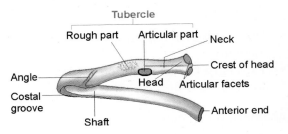

Fig. 5.8: Typical rib as seen from posterior aspect

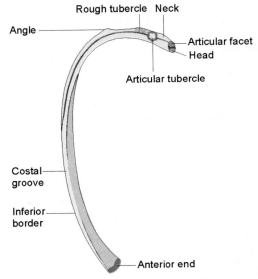

Fig. 5.9: Typical rib as seen from inferior aspect

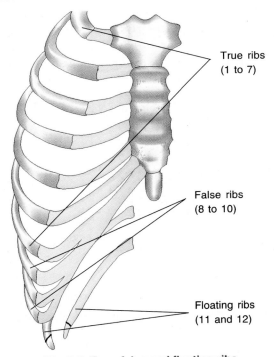

Fig. 5.7: True, false and floating ribs

is present at posterior end and bears one or two articular facets. The tubercle is a knob like structure present at the junction of the neck and shaft. The shaft is long and curved. The convex surface is the external surface while the concave surface is the internal surface, which bears a groove called as *subcostal groove*. The upper border of the shaft is rounded while lower border is sharp. The sternal end bears a concave depression for attachment of costal cartilage.

Side Determination

- The end of the rib having head, neck and tubercle (posterior end) should be kept posteriorly.
- The concave curved surface should be kept medially.
- The sharp border (inferior border) of the shaft should be kept downwards.

Anatomical Position

- The posterior end should be kept near the midline.
- The posterior end is at a higher level as compared to the anterior end.

General Features

The Posterior or Vertebral End

It includes head, neck and tubercle.
- The head presents two articular facets separated by the *crest of head* (Fig. 5.8). The lower facet is large and articulates with the body of the numerically corresponding vertebra. The upper small articular facet articulates with the body of the adjacent upper vertebra. The crest of the head is connected to the intervertebral disc by intra-articular ligament.

- The neck is short and has a sharp upper border. It is sometimes called as crest of the neck. The neck has an anterior smooth and a posterior rough surface.
- On the posterior aspect of the rib, just lateral to the neck, there is presence of an elevation called as tubercle. The tubercle has a medial articular (smooth) and lateral non-articular (rough) part.

The Anterior End

The anterior end of the rib has a cup shaped depression for articulation with the lateral end of the corresponding costal (smooth) cartilage to form *costochondral joint*.

The Shaft

The shaft of a typical rib is thin, flat and curved. It forms the major part of the rib. It extends between the tubercle and the anterior end of the rib.
- It has a superior rounded border and a sharp inferior border. It has an outer convex and an inner concave surface (Fig. 5.10).

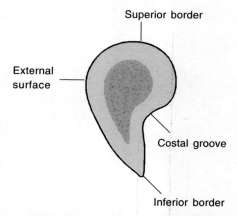

Fig. 5.10: Cross-section passing through shaft of a typical rib

- The inner surface shows a shallow *costal groove* just above the inferior border.
- The costal groove is well defined in the middle part of the shaft.
- A short distance lateral to the tubercle rib bends anteriorly. This is called as *posterior angle*.
- The rib also shows a twisting, because of which, two ends of the rib cannot touch a horizontal plane simultaneously (when kept on table).

Particular Features

Joints in Relation to the Typical Rib

- The head of a typical rib articulates with the adjacent vertebral bodies (with the numerically corresponding body and a body above it) and intervertebral disc to form *costovertebral joint* (Fig. 5.11A).
- The *costotransverse joint* is formed between the costal facet on the transverse process and the articular part of the tubercle (Fig. 5.11B).
- This joint is supported by various *costotransverse ligaments*, i.e., the lateral costotransverse, superior costotransverse and costotransverse ligaments.

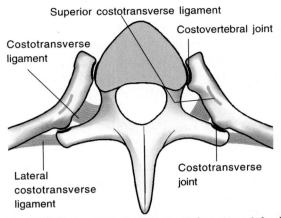

Fig. 5.11B: The costotransverse and costovertebral joints

The Muscles Attached on the Rib

- The attachments of *external intercostal*, *internal intercostal* and *innermost intercostal* are shown in Fig. 5.12.

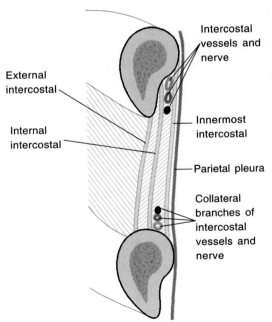

Fig. 5.12: The attachment of muscles between two adjacent ribs. In transverse section, as seen from superficial to deeper aspect

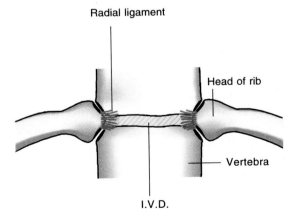

Fig. 5.11A: The costovertebral joint

- The various muscles are also attached on the external surface of the ribs, i.e., *pectoralis minor, serratus anterior, latissimus dorsi* and *back muscles.*
- The parietal pleura is related to the inner surface of the rib.

Nerves and Vessels Related to the Typical Rib

- The sympathetic trunk descends downwards on the anterior aspect of the heads of the typical ribs.
- The intercostal nerve and vessels lie in costal groove between internal intercostals and innermost intercostal muscles (Fig. 5.12).

The Atypical Ribs

The First Rib

The first rib is shortest, broadest, curved and flat rib (Fig. 5.13). As compared to the typical ribs its head has only one articular facet for the body of the first thoracic vertebra. The posterior angle of the rib lies at the tubercle itself. The shaft shows inner and outer borders thus superior and inferior surfaces.

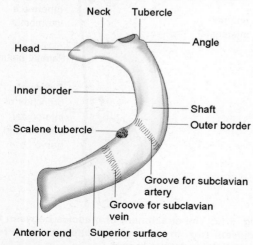

Fig. 5.13: First rib as seen from superior aspect

(This is in contrast to the typical ribs, which show superior and inferior borders and outer and inner surfaces.) The superior surface of the first rib is rough and shows the presence of two grooves. The inferior surface is smooth and there is absence of subcostal groove.

Side Determination

- The head, neck and tubercle are located posteriorly near the midline.
- The broad anterior end lies anteriorly.
- The concave inner border lies medially.
- The rough superior surface of the shaft (having grooves) should face superiorly.

Anatomical Position

- Keep the posterior or vertebral end near the midline.
- The anterior end is at the lower level as compared to the posterior end. In this position the upper surface should face anterosuperiorly.

General Features

The Posterior End

- The posterior end consists of head, neck and tubercle. The head is rounded, small and bears only one circular articular facet.
- The neck is rounded and extends upwards and posterolaterally.
- The neck shows superior, posterior, inferior and anterior surfaces.
- The tubercle is large and prominent. The oval articular facet on the tubercle articulates with the transverse process of first thoracic vertebra.

The Shaft

- The shaft is flat and shows superior and inferior surfaces and outer and inner borders.

- The superior surface of the first rib shows two shallow but wide grooves separated by a faint ridge. This ridge is continuous medially with the *scalene tubercle* on the inner border.
- The inferior surface is smooth and related to the parietal (costal) pleura.

Particular Features

Attachments of the Muscles on the First Rib (Fig. 5.14)

- The subclavius muscle arises from the superior surface near its anterior end.
- The scalenus anterior is inserted on the scalene tubercle. The scalenus medius is attached behind the groove for subclavian artery.
- The intercostal muscles arise from its outer border.
- The first digitation of the serratus anterior arises from its outer border.

Relations of the Nerves, Vessels and Ligaments (Fig. 5.14)

- The *costoclavicular ligament* is attached on its superior surface near its anterior end.

- The inner border gives attachment to the *suprapleural membrane.*
- The groove anterior to the scalene tubercle lodges the *subclavian vein.*
- The groove posterior to the scalene tubercle lodges *subclavian artery* and *lower trunk of the brachial plexus.*
- The anterior surface of the neck is related from medial to lateral side to: *sympathetic trunk, first posterior intercostal vein, superior intercostal artery and ascending branch of the ventral ramus of the first thoracic nerve.*

The Second Rib

The second rib is almost twice the length of first rib (Fig. 5.15A). The shaft has an external surface directed laterally and slightly upwards. This surface presents a prominent rough area near the middle of the shaft. It has a faint, short costal groove in the posterior part of the internal surface, which is directed downwards and medially.

Particular Features

- The prominent rough area on the outer surface, just behind the middle of the

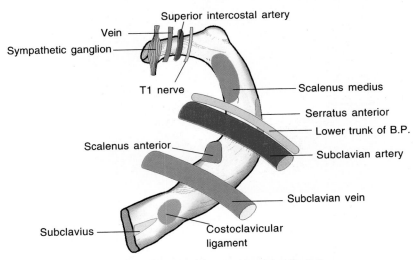

Fig. 5.14: Particular features of the first rib

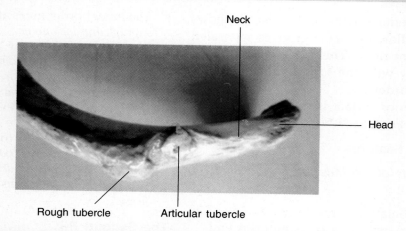

Fig. 5C: Medial end and inferior aspect of right typical rib. Note the head, neck and rough and smooth parts of tubercle

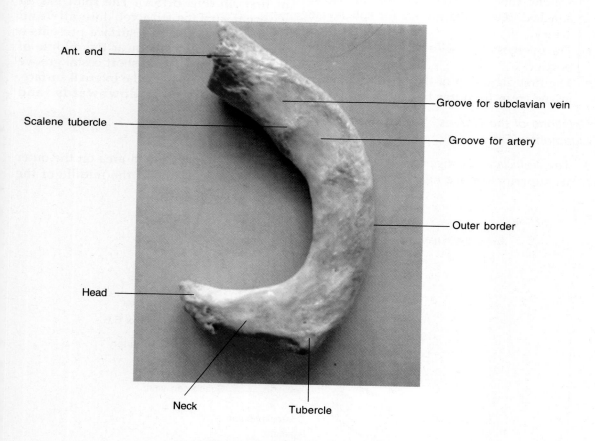

Fig. 5D: Superior surface of right first rib

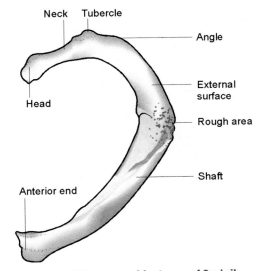

Fig. 5.15A: The general features of 2nd rib

The Tenth Rib

It also presents head, neck, tubercle, posterior angle and shaft, like a typical rib. However, it differs from typical ribs because it presents a single articular facet on its head for articulation with the 10th thoracic vertebral body.

The Eleventh Rib

This rib is short as compared to the tenth rib. It has no neck or tubercle. Its lateral end is tapering while vertebral end bears a single articular facet for the body of the eleventh thoracic vertebra.

The Twelfth Rib

- The twelfth rib is shorter than eleventh.
- It is directed downwards, laterally and forwards.
- Similar to eleventh rib it has no neck or tubercle (Fig. 5.16).
- It has no angle and there is also the absence of subcostal groove.
- It has a single facet on head for articulation with the body of 12th thoracic vertebra.
- It has a pointed lateral end, which gives attachment to cartilage.
- This rib presents upper and lower borders and anterior and posterior surfaces.

shaft, gives origin to the 1st and 2nd digitations of the serratus anterior (Fig. 5.15B).

- The outer surface in its posterior part gives insertion to the scalenus posterior muscle.
- The intercostal muscle are attached on its upper and lower borders.

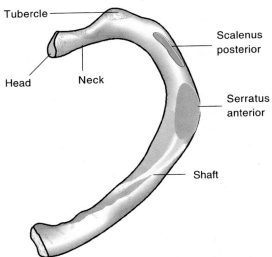

Fig. 5.15B: The second rib showing attachment of muscles

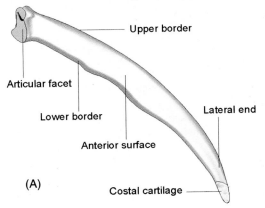

(A)

(B)

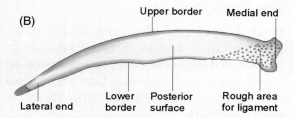

Figs. 5.16A and B: The general features of 12th rib, (A) Anterior aspect, (B) Posterior aspect

- The anterior surface is smooth and concave and faces slightly upwards.

Particular Features of 12th Rib

- The medial part of the upper border gives attachment to the intercostal muscles (Fig. 5.17A).
- The lateral part of the upper border gives attachment to the diaphragm.
- The quadratus lumborum muscle with its covering (anterior layer of the thoraco-lumbar fascia) is attached on the medial half of the anterior surface.
- The transverse abdominis muscle is attached on the lower lateral part of the anterior surface.

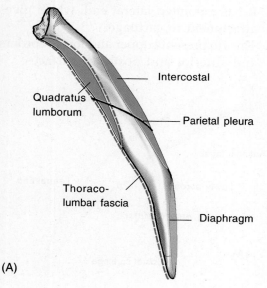

(A)

(B)

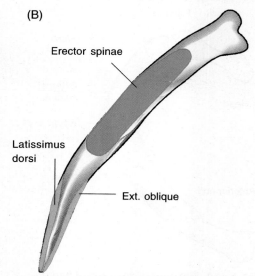

Fig. 5.17: The particular features of 12th rib as seen from (A) front and (B) behind

- The lower limit of the parietal (costal) pleura crosses the anterior surface of rib and quadratus lumborum muscle. Thus costodiaphragmatic recess extends on the anterior aspect of the medial half of the rib.
- The attachments of the muscles on the posterior aspect of the twelfth rib are shown in Fig. 5.17B.

Ossification of Rib

A typical rib is ossified from one primary and three secondary centers (one for head and two for tubercle) (Fig. 5.18). Primary and secondary centers fuse after 20 years of age.

The Costal Cartilages

- The costal cartilages are flattened bars of hyaline cartilage.
- They prolong the ribs anteriorly (Fig. 5.7).
- Each costal cartilage has anterior and posterior surfaces and upper and lower borders.

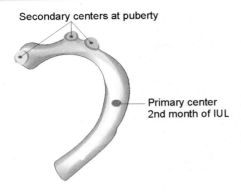

Secondary centers at puberty

Primary center
2nd month of IUL

Fig. 5.18: Ossification of a typical rib

- The first seven costal cartilages join to sternum.
- The 8th, 9th and 10th articulate with the cartilage just superior to them. The 11th and 12th costal cartilages form caps on the anterior end of these ribs.
- The length of costal cartilages increases from the first to the seventh. The length decreases gradually from 8th to the 12th.
- The costal cartilage provides elasticity and mobility to the thoracic wall.
- They prevent fractures of sternum and ribs due to their resilience.

CLINICAL IMPORTANCE

Fractures of Ribs

When there occurs a direct injury on the sidewall of the chest, the broken ends of the ribs may tear pleura and lung. This may lead to the collection of air (pneumothorax) or blood (haemothorax) in the pleural cavity.

When there is indirect violence, due to compression of the chest against steering wheel in accidents, ribs are commonly fractured near their angles.

Ribs are Used for Bone Grafting

Similar to the fibula ribs are also used for bone grafting. In this procedure, the periosteum of the rib is incised along its length and a segment of the rib is removed for grafting leaving the periosteum intact. After some time, rib regenerates deep to the periosteum.

Extra Ribs

Sometimes the number of ribs may increase (than normal 12 pairs) due to the presence of a cervical or lumbar rib.

The cervical rib articulates with the 7th cervical vertebra but usually fails to attach to the sternum. The anterior end of the cervical rib may attach to the first rib. The cervical rib may compress the lower trunk of the brachial plexus. This may lead to pain and numbness in the shoulder and upper limb. This rib may also compress the subclavian artery resulting in pain in the upper limb due to poor blood supply to the limb muscles.

Lumbar ribs are less common as compared to the cervical ribs.

THORACIC VERTEBRAE

The thoracic part of the vertebral column is formed by the twelve thoracic vertebrae and intervertebral discs. This part of the column is concave anteriorly (refer Fig. 4.1).

Thoracic vertebrae are larger and stronger than cervical vertebrae. Compared to the cervical vertebrae they also have longer and larger transverse processes. The following three special features are helpful in the identification of thoracic vertebrae.

- Presence of costal facets or demi-facets on the bodies for articulation with the heads of the ribs.
- Presence of costal facets on their transverse processes for articulation with the tubercle of the ribs (except for T11 and T12 vertebrae).
- The spinous processes of T3 to T9 vertebrae are long and slopes downwards. The spinous process of T11 and

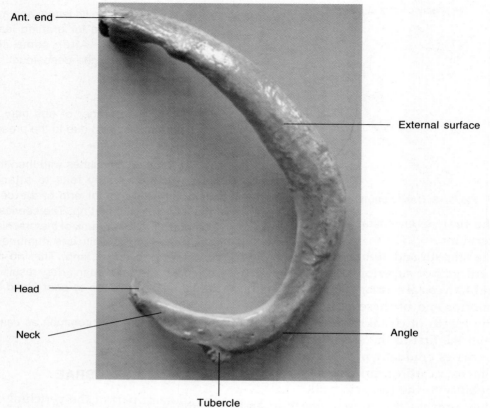

Ant. end

External surface

Head

Neck

Angle

Tubercle

Fig. 5E: Superior surface of right second rib

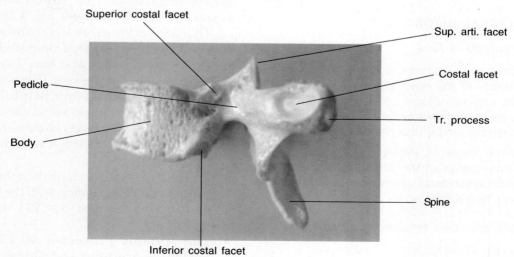

Superior costal facet

Sup. arti. facet

Costal facet

Pedicle

Tr. process

Body

Spine

Inferior costal facet

Fig. 5F: Left lateral view of a typical thoracic vertebra

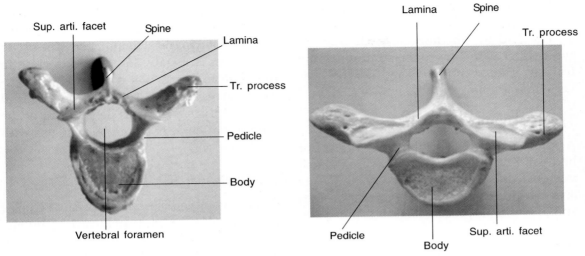

Fig. 5G: Superior aspect of a typical thoracic vertebra

Fig. 5H: Superior aspect of the first thoracic vertebra

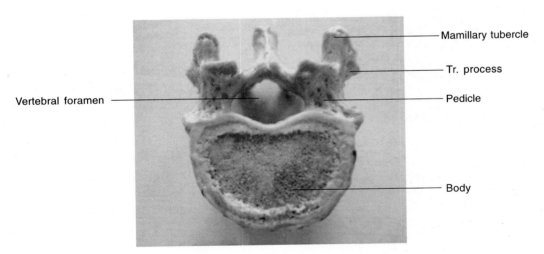

Fig. 5I: Superior aspect of 12th thoracic vertebra

T12 are shorter, broader and directed more posteriorly.

The 2nd to 9th thoracic vertebrae are typical because they bear common bony features. The 1st, 10th 11th and 12th thoracic vertebrae are atypical.

Typical Thoracic Vertebrae

A typical thoracic vertebra is made up of body and neural arch (vertebral arch). Each vertebra has seven processes, i.e., four articular processes, two transverse processes and one spinous process (Figs. 5.19 and 5.20).

Body

The superior and inferior surfaces of the body of a typical vertebra are heart shaped (Fig. 5.19). The lateral aspect of body, close to its upper and lower borders, shows the presence of two costal demi-facets. The upper demi-facet is usually larger and is close to the pedicle. It articulates with the numerically corresponding rib. The lower costal demi-facet is smaller and lies in front of the inferior vertebral notch and articulates with the lower rib.

Vertebral Arch

It consists of pedicles and laminae. Pedicles are short and directed backwards. Laminae are short, thick and flat vertical plates of the bone that join in midline to form the posterior portion of the vertebral arch. The superior vertebral notch is shallow and present above the pedicle while inferior vertebral notch is deep and present below the pedicle (Fig. 5.20). The vertebral foramen is small and circular. It is bounded by body, pedicles and laminae.

Processes

The transverse processes are large, club shaped and directed laterally and somewhat backwards. On their anterior surface they bear oval costal facet for articulation with the tubercle of the rib (costotransverse articulation). The costal facets on the upper six transverse processes are concave and directed anterolaterally. While the costal facets in 7th to 10th transverse processes are flat and directed upwards, forwards and laterally.

The superior articular facets are directed posterolaterally while the inferior articular facets are directed anteromedially.

The spinous processes are long and directed downwards.

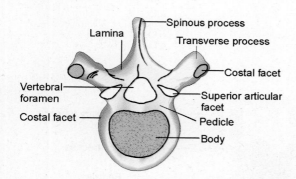

Fig. 5.19: A typical thoracic vertebra as seen from above

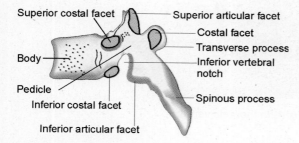

Fig. 5.20: A typical thoracic vertebra as seen from lateral side

Atypical Thoracic Vertebra

First Thoracic Vertebra

Following features will help to identify the first thoracic vertebra (Fig. 5.21):

- The body is like cervical vertebrae, i.e., its anteroposterior diameter is less than its transverse diameter.
- There is presence of a single circular costal facet on the lateral surface of the body for articulation with the head of the first rib.
- Presence of a small costal demi-facet near its lower border for articulation with the upper demi-facet on the head of 2nd rib.
- The vertebral foramen is large and triangular (similar to the cervical vertebra).
- Spinous process is long and directed backwards.

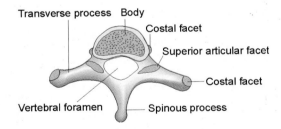

Fig. 5.21: First thoracic vertebra as seen from superior aspect

Tenth Thoracic Vertebra

- The shape of the body is somewhat like lumbar vertebrae.
- Mostly it bears a single circular costal facet for the head of the 10th rib (Fig. 5.22). It means the head of the 10th rib will not articulate with the body of 9th thoracic vertebra. Hence the body of 9th vertebra will have only upper demi-facet.

- The costal facet is present on the anterior aspect of the transverse process for the tubercle of 10th rib.

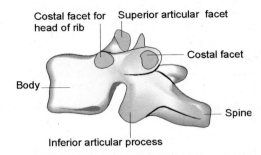

Fig. 5.22: The lateral aspect of 10th thoracic vertebra. Note the directions of superior and inferior articular facets, they are typical thoracic type

Eleventh Thoracic Vertebra

- Body is large and somewhat lumbar type.
- A single circular costal facet on the lateral aspect of the body.
- The transverse process is short and bears no costal facet, as 11th rib is a floating rib.
- The superior and inferior articular facets are thoracic type. (Sometimes inferior articular facet may be lumbar type).
- The spinous process may be somewhat like a lumbar vertebra.

Twelfth Thoracic Vertebra

- Body is large and lumbar type (kidney shaped).
- The single circular costal facet for the head of the 12th rib. The facet is present mid way between upper and lower borders and tends to encroach on the lateral aspect of the pedicle (Fig. 5.23).
- Similar to the 11th vertebra there is absence of costal facet on the transverse process.
- The transverse processes of T12 are short (rudimentary) and presents three

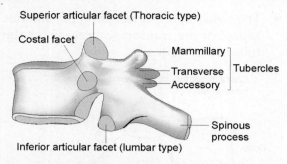

Fig. 5.23: Twelfth thoracic vertebra as seen from lateral side

tubercles, i.e., superior, inferior and lateral. The lateral tubercle represents true transverse process.

- The inferior articular facets are lumbar like, i.e., they are convex and face antero-laterally. The superior articular facets are thoracic type, i.e., flat and directed posterolaterally.

- The spinous process is also like a lumbar vertebra, i.e., short, broad and directed backwards.

Articulation of a Typical Rib with the Vertebrae (Costovertebral and Costotransverse Joints)

A typical rib articulates posteriorly with the bodies of two adjacent vertebrae and the transverse process of the lower vertebra (Fig. 5.24). Students should practice this articulation with the help of two typical thoracic vertebrae and a typical rib.

The Costovertebral Joint

The head of the rib bears two demi-facets. The upper small demi-facet articulates with the body of the adjacent upper vertebra. The crest of the head (which is present between two demi-facets) is connected to the intervertebral disc by interarticular ligament. The lower larger demi-facet on the head of the rib articulates with the body of the numerically corresponding vertebra (Fig. 5.11A).

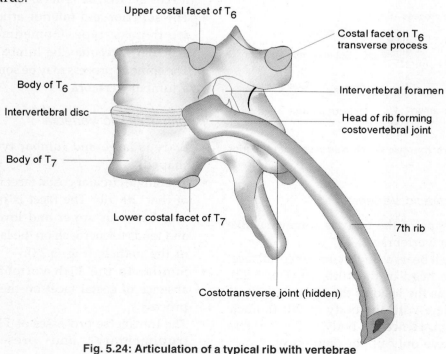

Fig. 5.24: Articulation of a typical rib with vertebrae

The Costotransverse Joint

The articular part of the tubercle of the rib presents an oval facet. It articulates with the articular facet on the transverse process of the corresponding vertebra (Fig. 5.11B).

This can be further understood by looking at the articulation of the 7th rib. The head of the 7th rib articulates with the body of 6th thoracic vertebra (with the demi-facet near its lower border) and with the body of 7th thoracic vertebra (with the demi-facet near its upper border). The head is also connected with the intervertebral disc between 6th and 7th thoracic vertebrae. The tubercle of the 7th rib also articulates with the transverse process of the 7th thoracic vertebra.

Ossification of Thoracic Vertebra

A typical thoracic vertebra ossifies by three primary centers, i.e., one for body and one for each neural arch. These centers unite with each other between 3 to 5 years of age (Fig. 5.25).

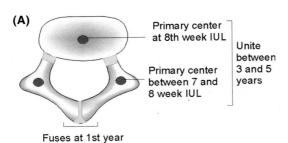

(A)

Primary center at 8th week IUL
Primary center between 7 and 8 week IUL
} Unite between 3 and 5 years

Fuses at 1st year

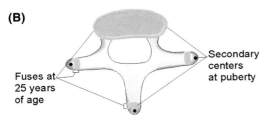

(B)

Fuses at 25 years of age
Secondary centers at puberty

Fig. 5.25: (A) Ossification by primary centers (B) Ossification by secondary centers

At puberty, five secondary centers appear, i.e., one for spine, one for each transverse process and two ring like centers at the margin of upper and lower surface of body.

CLINICAL IMPORTANCE

Tuberculosis of Thoracic Vertebrae

Spongy bone in the body of thoracic vertebrae is the most common site of tubercular infection. Tubercular bacilli reach the spongy bone through blood circulation and settle there due to sluggish blood flow and restricted mobility of thoracic coloumn.

The infection leads to the destruction of spongy bone and production of "Cold pus". As the chronic injection of tubercle bacilli does not produce the local sign of heat, pain and redness, it is called as cold abscess. Due to destruction of spongy bone body is collapsed resulting in the production of kyphosis.

Scoliosis and Kyphosis

Thracic coloumn is the most common site where scoliosis and kyphosis is produced (See Further Details). Kyphosis is most commonly seen in old age due to weakness of spongy bone of vertebral bodies (Osteoporosis).

Hemivertebra

Sometimes the body of vertebra ossify by two primary centers, one for each lateral half of the body. If one of these centers fails to ossify then only half of vertebral body is formed. This leads to the lateral bending of column on one side.

FURTHER DETAILS

Biomechanics of the Thoracic Cage

Ribs play an important role in the stability of thoracic spine. The study of Andriacchi et al. (1974) indicated that the stiffness of the thoracic spine was greatly enhanced by the presence of rib cage. The stiffness of spine, with ribs and sternum was found to be 2.5 times that of ligamentous spine alone. Removal of the sternum from the rib cage completely destroys the stiffness of the thoracic column.

On the basis of morphometric studies on thoracic vertebrae, Pal and Routal (1987), could find that ribs are involved in transmission of considerable magnitude of load from sternum to vertebrae. Load on the rib is expected to come from various sources. Ribs carry weight of thoracic wall, i.e., weight of muscles attached to thoracic wall including intercostal muscles, parietal pleura and weight of ribs and sternum itself. In case of females the load of breast is also carried through ribs. Since the lower ribs give attachment to diaphragm the weight of upper abdominal viscera, in part, is also expected to be transmitted through ribs. However, most important of all of these is transmission of weight of upper limbs. Forces from upper limbs are brought to the sternum through clavicles. From here it is carried through sternum to ribs.

The role of ribs in load transmission was investigated by Pal (1989) on the basis of mechanical considerations, morphometric and spongy trabecular bone studies. It was revealed that different ribs transmitted different magnitude of force from sternum to the vertebral column. The first, 6th and 7th ribs transmitted maximum force while rib number 2, 3 and 4 transmitted minimum.

The above studies also confirmed the route of load transmission from sternum to the vertebral column. From the rib the load reaches the body and intervertebral disc through costovertebral joint. But a part of the load also reaches the corresponding lamina through costotransverse articulation and transverse process. From the lamina the load passes to the next vertebra through facet joint and ultimately reaches the body of this vertebra through its pedicle (Fig. 5.26).

This route was confirmed on the basis of strong correlation between rib circumference, lamina index (width × thickness of lamina) and pedicle index (height × width of pedicle) at each vertebral level, as these parameters indicate the relative magnitude of load passing through them.

A study by Routal and Pal (1990) revealed two important facts:

1. The 65% of the total force passing through a rib was transmitted via head (costovertebral joint) and 35% through the articular facet of the tubercle (costotransverse joint).

2. Significant bilateral symmetry was observed in the transmission of forces on both sides.

The stability of thoracic column in normal conditions is maintained because of equal force brought by the ribs from both sides (Routal and Pal, 1990). An asymmetric load transmission through the ribs may lead to compression of facet joint and intervertebral disc on the side which transmits more force.

Above findings were the basis for generation of a hypothesis for the mechanism of production

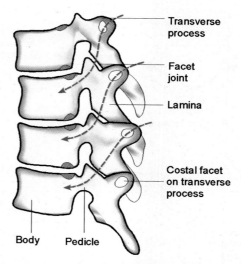

Fig. 5.26: Lateral aspect of a part of thoracic column. Arrows indicate the route of the weight transmission from ribs to the bodies of the lower vertebrae

of scolioses (Pal, 1990). According to which the vertical stability of the thoracic spine is maintained by equal support provided by ribs from both sides. At each vertebral level, equal support is provided due to the equal weight brought to posterior column (laminae) from two sides through the ribs. The intervertebral joints at each level (between bodies and articular processes) can be considered as the fulcrum of a balance resting on three points (body and two facets) and the rib on either side as two arms of a balance (Fig. 15.27).

Any interference in this balancing mechanism will disturb the mechanism of spinal stability. Spine will bend towards the heavier side at the intervertebral joints.

The above hypothesis has been confirmed by experiments on rabbits (Pal et al., 1991 and Pal et al., 1993).

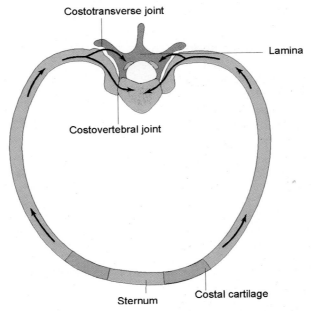

Fig. 5.27: Schematic diagram showing the transmission of force from sternum to vertebral column through ribs. The 65% of total load passing through each rib is transmitted via costovertebral joint and 35% through costotransverse joint

Further Readings

- Andriacchi T.P. et al. (1974). *Journal of Biomechanics* 7, 497-506.
- Jit I., Jhingan V. and Kulkarni M. (1980) Am. J. of Phys. Anthrop 53: 217-224.
- Pal G.P. and Routal R.V. (1987). *Journal of Anatomy* (London) 152, 93-106.
- Pal G.P. (1989). *Journal of A.S.I.* 38(3), 145-161.

- Pal G.P. (1990). *Spine* (Am. Vol.) 16, 288-292.
- Pal G.P., Bhatt R.H. and Patel V.S. (1991) *Spine* (Am. Vol.) 16, 137-142.
- Pal G.P. et al. (1993). *Journal of A.S.I.*, 42, 105-144.
- Routal R.V. and Pal G.P. (1990) *J. of A.S.I.* 39 (2), 153-160.

6) Bones of the Abdominal and Pelvic Regions

The bones of the abdominal region consist of five lumbar vertebrae and intervening intervertebral discs. The bones of the pelvic region consist of two hip bones (right and left), sacrum and coccyx. The right and left hip bones are joined anteriorly at the pubic symphysis and to the sacrum posteriorly to form *bony pelvis.*

We shall first study the lumbar vertebrae, sacrum and coccyx before studying the bony pelvis. Students are advised to review the features of a typical vertebra (as described in Chapter 4), before studying lumbar vertebrae.

LUMBAR VERTEBRAE

The lumbar region of the vertebral column consists of five lumbar vertebrae. The upper four vertebrae are typical while the fifth is atypical.

Features of a Typical Lumbar Vertebra

Body

The bodies of lumbar vertebrae are large and kidney shaped (Fig. 6.1A). The size of the lumbar vertebrae increases from above downwards as they have to bear the increasing weight of the body.

Pedicles

The pedicles are short and strong. They are directed backwards and somewhat laterally. The superior vertebral notches are shallow while inferior notches are deep (Fig. 6.1B).

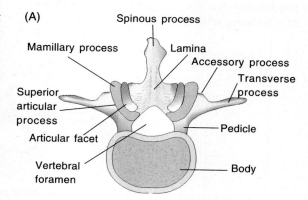

(A)

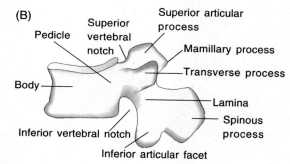

(B)

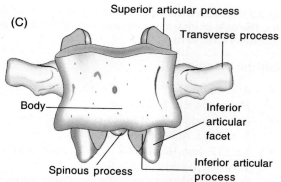

(C)

Fig. 6.1: A typical lumbar vertebra as seen from (A) above, from (B) lateral aspect and from (C) front

Lamina

These are broad and short and do not overlap one another as in case of thoracic vertebrae.

Vertebral Foramen

The vertebral foramen is large in size and vary in shape, i.e., oval (L1) to triangular (L4).

Transverse Processes

These are thin, long and often have tapering end. The posteroinferior aspect of the root of each transverse process bears a small projection called as *accessory process*.

Superior Articular Processes

These are vertical curved processes and bear concave articular facet facing backward and medially. There is the presence of a non-articular rough projection on the posterior border of the superior articular process called as *mammillary process*.

Inferior Articular Processes

These are also vertical processes. They bear convex articular facet, which is directed forwards and laterally (Fig. 6.1C).

Spinous Process

The spinous process of a typical vertebra is large, thick, horizontal and quadrilateral in shape. It presents thickened posterior and inferior borders.

Features of Fifth Lumbar Vertebra

- The fifth lumbar vertebra is the largest of all the vertebrae. The body and transverse processes of L5 are very massive (Fig. 6.2) as they carry the weight of whole upper body.

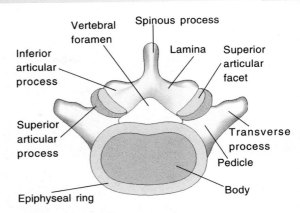

Fig. 6.2: Superior view of fifth lumbar vertebra

- The vertical height of the anterior surface of body is more as compared to the posterior surface. This fact is responsible for a prominent sacrovertebral angle (angle between long axis of lumbar column and long axis of sacrum).
- The transverse processes of L5 are very large and thick. They have a wide origin, i.e., they arise from the lateral aspect of pedicle and also encroaches on the side of the body. The transverse processes of L5 are massive because they are involved in transmission of load from the body of L5 to the ilium (through ilio-lumbar ligament) and to the sacrum (through lumbo-sacral ligament).
- The spinous process of L5 vertebra is short and directed backwards and somewhat downwards.
- The distance between two superior articular processes is almost equal to the distance between two inferior articular processes. (In case of a typical lumbar vertebra the distance between two superior articular processes is more as compared to distance between two inferior processes (Fig. 6.3).

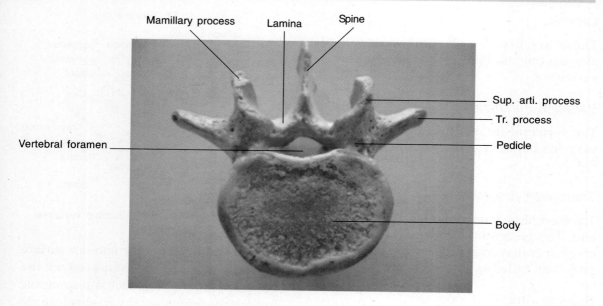

Fig. 6A: Superior aspect of the typical lumbar vertebra

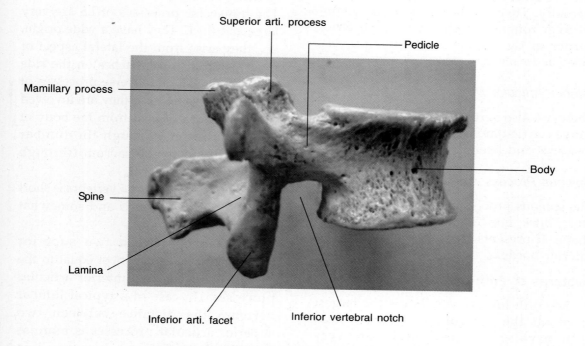

Fig. 6B: Right lateral view of a typical lumbar vertebra

Lamina   Vertebral foramen

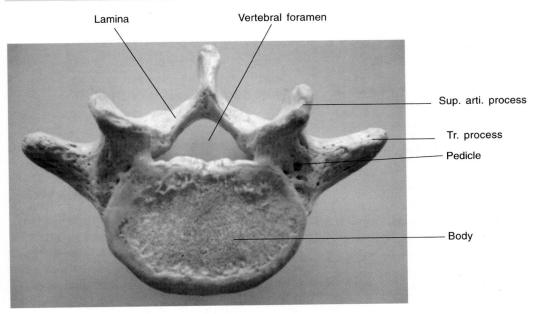

Sup. arti. process

Tr. process

Pedicle

Body

Fig. 6C: Superior aspect of 5th lumbar vertebra

Tr. process

Sup. arti. process   Body

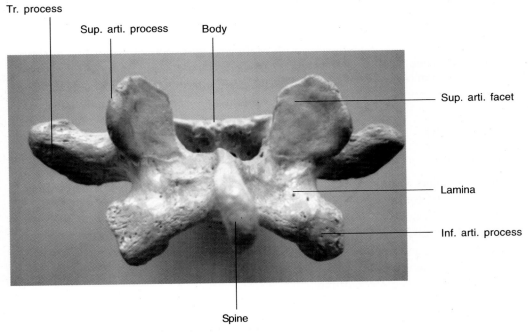

Sup. arti. facet

Lamina

Inf. arti. process

Spine

Fig. 6D: Posterior aspect of the 5th lumbar vertebra

(A)

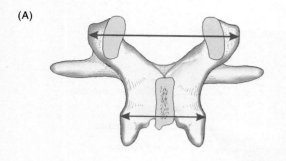

(B)

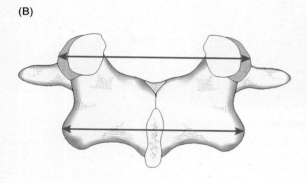

Fig. 6.3: Distance between two superior and two inferior articular processes of (A) typical and (B) fifth lumbar vertebra

---

CLINICAL APPLICATION

Lumbar Spinal Stenosis

In this condition there occurs the narrowing of the lumbar part of the vertebral canal. The condition may result due to bulging (prolapse) of intervertebral disc, arthritic proliferation or ligamentous degeneration. Sometimes stenosis may be congenital also. The stenosis causes compression of the spinal nerve roots of the cauda equina. The condition is usually treated surgically by laminectomy (excision of vertebral laminae) or by removing entire vertebral arch.

Low Back Pain

The neural arch at L4 and L5 levels is involved in transmission of a considerable magnitude of load. This fact indicates that the joints between the articular facets may be site for low back pain. Probably, the pain is due to stretching of the joint capsule (or transmission of load across it), which contains a nociceptive type IV receptor system (Pal and Routal, 1987).

Instability of Spine Following Laminectomy

About 20% of load in the lumbar region passes through laminae of lumbar vertebrae. Thus the laminectomy leads to instability of lumbar column. Pal and Routal (1987) strongly recommended the preservation of the integrity of the articular facet joints in laminectomy.

Spondylolysis and Spondylolisthesis

Refer Chapter 4.

Prolapsed or Herniated Disc

A prolapsed disc occurs when the nucleus pulposus pushes outward, distorting the shape of the disc. If the annulus fibrosus of the disc ruptures (usually on posterolateral aspect and most commonly at L4/L5 or L5/S1 levels) then the nucleus pulposus is herniated through the rupture. Both in prolapsed or herniated disc surrounding tissue become inflamed and swollen. The tissue of the disc may press on the nerve or spinal cord, causing pain e.g. sciatica.

THE SACRUM

The sacrum is composed of five fused sacral vertebrae in adults. It is a large, triangular wedge shaped bone (Fig. 6.4). It is wedged between two hip bones and forms the posterior part of bony pelvis. It transmits the

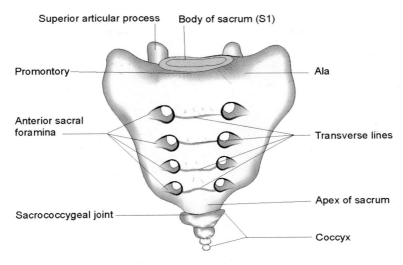

Fig. 6.4: The anterior (pelvic) surface of sacrum

weight of upper body received through L5 to the pelvic girdle through sacroiliac joints. The sacrum is triangular because there is rapid decrease in size of the lower sacrum. This is due to the fact that lower sacrum (the portion below the sacroiliac joint) is not involved in weight bearing hence its size diminishes rapidly.

The triangular sacrum presents an upper end or base (Fig. 6.5). The base is formed by the superior surface of S1 vertebra. It articulates with the fifth lumbar vertebra at lumbosacral joint. The lower end of sacrum is tapering and also known as apex. It articulates with the coccyx. Sacrum presents

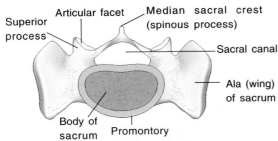

Fig. 6.5: The superior surface (base) of sacrum (S1 vertebra)

an anterior (or pelvic) concave surface (Fig. 6.4) and a dorsal (or posterior) convex surface (Fig. 6.6). The pelvic surface shows the presence of four pairs of *anterior sacral foramina*. Similarly, the posterior surface also shows four pairs of *posterior sacral foramina*. The sacrum also presents right and left lateral surfaces that articulate with the iliac part of the right and left hip bones to form *sacroiliac joints* (Fig. 6.7).

The *sacral canal* is the continuation of the vertebral canal in the sacrum. The canal lies posterior to the median part of the sacrum formed by fused bodies. The sacral canal communicates with the anterior and posterior sacral foramina through which passes the ventral and dorsal rami of sacral nerves.

Anatomical Position

Hold the bone in such a way that the pelvic (anterior) surface is directed forwards and downwards. In this situation the base of the sacrum will look forward and upwards.

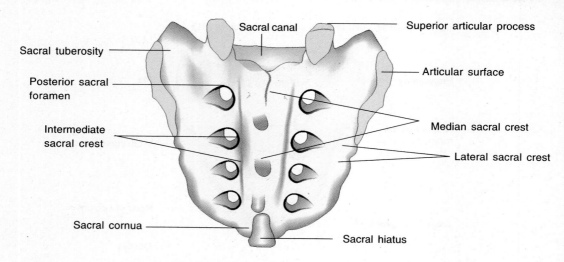

Sacral tuberosity

Posterior sacral foramen

Intermediate sacral crest

Sacral cornua

Sacral canal

Superior articular process

Articular surface

Median sacral crest

Lateral sacral crest

Sacral hiatus

Fig. 6.6: The posterior surface of sacrum

General Features

Base of the Sacrum

It is formed by the upper surface of the first sacral vertebra. The base consists of a centrally placed oval body and upper surface of right and left ala (lateral mass) on each side of the body (Fig. 6.5). Posterior to the body there is the presence of triangular sacral canal bounded by thick pedicles and laminae. The superior articular facets project upwards from the junction of the pedicles and laminae. The superior articular facets of the sacrum articulate with the inferior articular facets of 5th lumbar vertebra. Posteriorly, there is presence of a tubercle at the meeting point of two laminae. This tubercle represents the rudimentary spinous process.

The body of the first sacral vertebra is large and much wider. Its anterior border is projecting and called the sacral promontory. The lateral portion of the base (ala of the sacrum) is smooth and like a wing. The ala of the sacrum is strong as it has to transmit the load from lumbosacral joint to the sacroiliac joint.

Pelvic (Anterior) Surface

This surface is smooth, concave and faces downwards and forwards. This surface presents four transverse lines indicating the site of fusion of 5 sacral vertebrae (Fig. 6.4). At the ends of these transverse lines there are four pairs of sacral foramina on this surface. These foramina communicate with the sacral canal through intervertebral foramina.

Posterior (Dorsal) Surface

The dorsal surface of the sacrum is rough and convex.

- In the mid line there is the presence of a longitudinal ridge called as *median sacral crest*, which is formed by the fused spinous processes of the upper four sacral vertebrae (Fig. 6.6).
- The dorsal surface presents four pairs of *dorsal sacral foramina*, which communicate with the sacral canal and transmit dorsal rami of upper four sacral spinous nerves.
- An area between right and left foramina is formed by the fusion of laminae of

upper four sacral vertebrae. The laminae of fifth sacral vertebra (and sometimes fourth also) fail to fuse in midline and presents an inverted U or V shaped gap called as *sacral hiatus.*

- On either side of the sacral hiatus are the sacral *cornua,* which represent the inferior articular processes of fifth sacral vertebra. The sacral hiatus contains fatty connective tissue, filum-terminale, the S5 nerve and coccygeal nerve. The sacral cornua can be easily palpated in a living person and are useful guide to locate the hiatus for injection of anesthetic agents.
- On medial side of dorsal sacral foramina is a vertical crest consisting of four small tubercles. These tubercles represent the fused articular processes of fused sacral vertebrae. This crest is called *intermediate crest.*
- On the lateral side of the dorsal sacral foramina there is the presence of *lateral sacral crest.* This crest is formed by the fusion of transverse processes.

Lateral Surface of the Sacrum

On both the lateral surfaces of the sacrum there is presence of a large ear shaped (Fig. 6.7) *auricular surface* that articulates with the ilium of each hip bone to form sacroiliac joint. Posterior to the auricular surface is rough area, the *sacral tuberosity* for attachment of strong *interosseous sacroiliac ligament.*

Apex of the Sacrum

It has an oval facet for articulation with the coccyx.

The Coccyx

It is a small triangular bone formed by the

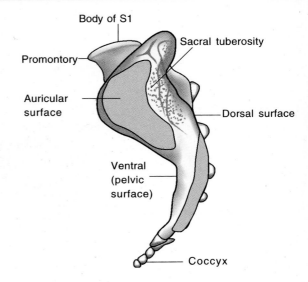

Fig. 6.7: Lateral surface of sacrum

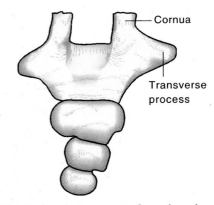

Fig. 6.8: The coccyx bone as seen from dorsal aspect

fusion of four rudimentary vertebrae (Fig. 6.8). It has an upper end (base), lower end and pelvic and dorsal surfaces. The base is formed by first coccygeal vertebra, which has an oval facet for articulation with the apex of the sacrum. The first coccygeal vertebra also has transverse processes and cornua. The cornua project upwards from the base of the coccyx and are connected with the cornua of

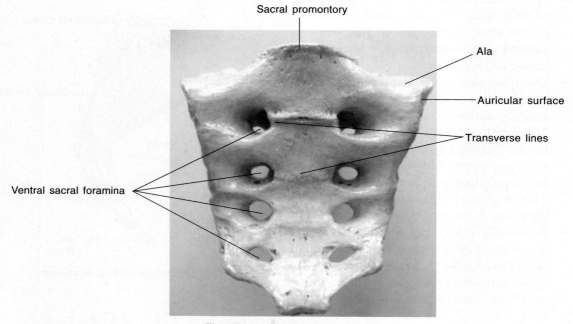

Fig. 6E: Anterior surface of sacrum

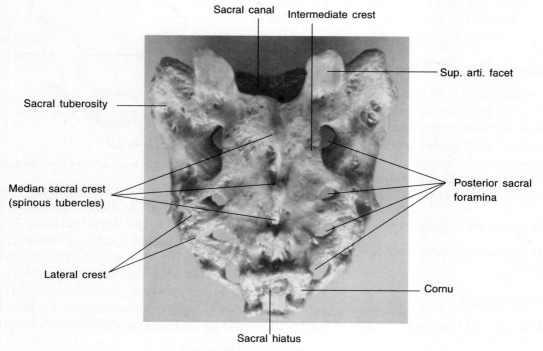

Fig. 6F: Posterior aspect of sacrum

the sacrum through ligaments. The remaining coccygeal vertebrae are featureless and represented by the nodules of bone.

Particular Features of the Sacrum and Coccyx

Attachments of the Muscles on the Sacrum and Coccyx

- Iliacus and piriformis muscles are attached on the pelvic surface of the sacrum (Fig. 6.9).
- The coccygeus muscle is inserted on the pelvic surface of 5th sacral vertebra and coccyx.
- The levator ani is inserted on the tip of coccyx.
- Note the origin of gluteus maximus from the sacrum and coccyx from their dorsal surfaces (Fig. 6.10).
- The dorsal surface also gives origin to the erector spinae and multifidus.

Attachment of Ligaments

- The *sacrotuberous ligament* is attached on lower part of dorsal surface of sacrum (Fig. 6.11).
- The lateral margin of lower part of sacrum and lateral margin of the coccyx give attachment to the *sacrospinous ligament*.
- The *interosseous ligament* of the sacrospinous joint is attached on the rough area on the lateral surface posterior to the auricular surface (Fig. 6.10).
- The iliolumbar ligament is attached to the lateral margin of ala and iliac crest.

Nerves and Blood Vessels in Relation to the Pelvic and Dorsal Surface of the Sacrum

- The median sacral artery is related in mid line (Fig. 6.9).

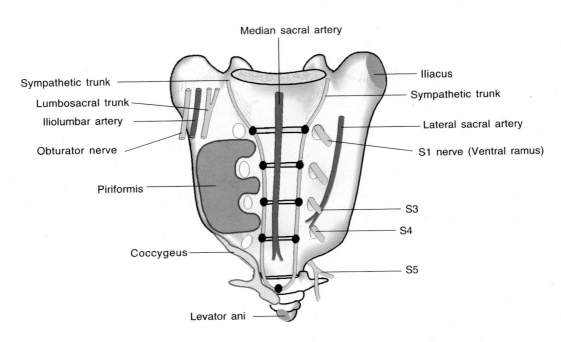

Fig. 6.9: The pelvic surface of sacrum showing the particular features

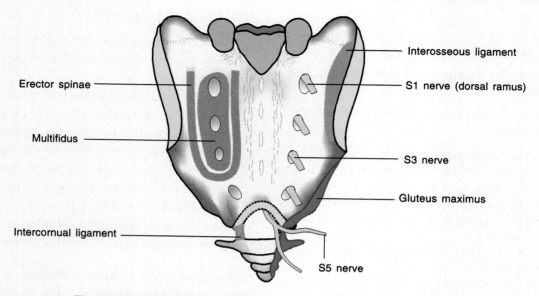

Fig. 6.10: The dorsal surface of sacrum showing the particular features

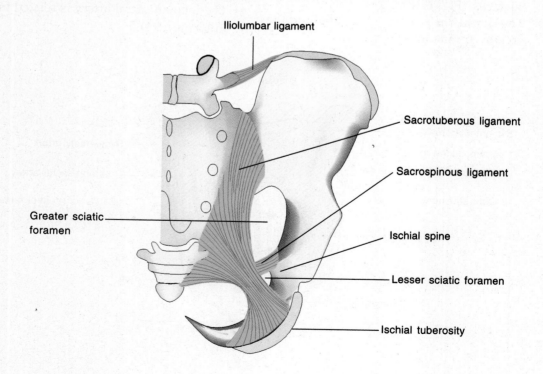

Fig. 6.11: Attachment of ligaments

- The lateral sacral artery is related lateral to the ventral sacral foramina.
- The right and left sympathetic trunks are related medial to the ventral sacral foramina (Fig. 6.9).
- The superior rectal artery is related to the left side of the midline.
- The dorsal and ventral sacral foramina give passage to the dorsal and ventral spinal rami respectively (Figs. 6.9 and 6.10).
- The sacral canal contains the *cauda equina*.
- The subdural and subarachnoid spaces end at the middle of the sacrum.
- Each ala of the sacrum is related to the following structures from medial to the lateral-sympathetic trunk, lumbosacral trunk, iliolumbar artery and obturator nerve (Fig. 6.9).

CLINICAL IMPORTANCE

Caudal Epidural Anesthesia

As the subdural and subarachnoid spaces end at the level of the middle of the sacrum, the sacral canal contains extradural or epidural space filled with fibro-fatty tissue. In this space there are spinal nerves of *cauda equina* covered by dura. In the *epidural anesthesia* (*caudal analgesia*) a local anesthetic agent is injected in sacral canal through the sacral hiatus. The sacral hiatus is located by palpating sacral cornua and lower end of median sacral crest. The anesthetic agent when injected in the sacral hiatus acts on the spinal nerves in the cauda equina (usually S2 to coccygeal nerves). This procedure is usually used to relax the perineal musculature for painless childbirth.

Abnormal Fusion of Lumbar and Sacral Vertebrae

Sometimes (in about 5% of people) L5 vertebra is partly or completely fused with the sacrum.

The condition is called as *sacralization* of L5 vertebra. In some cases, S1 vertebra is separated from sacrum and may be partly or completely separated from sacrum. This condition is called as *lumbarization* of S1 vertebra. Both the above conditions may produce painful symptoms in persons having abnormal fusion of the vertebra.

FURTHER DETAILS

Weight Transmission Through the Sacrum

An attempt has been made by Pal (1989) to find the route and relative magnitude of weight passing through different components of the sacrum. It was found that out of total forces acting on the body and two articular facets, at upper end of sacrum, 67% passes through body, 21% through two articular facets and 12% passes directly from the transverse processes of fifth lumbar vertebra to the ala of sacrum through the lumbosacral ligament.

Since 21% of the total load is borne by the articular facets, in the absence of one or both of the facets this load is likely to reach the sacrum through the accessory articulation between the ala and transverse process of the fifth lumbar vertebra. It was observed that in specimens where the articular facet was absent on one or both sides, there was always an accessory facet on the ala of the sacrum so that the load was transmitted to the ala from the transverse process of the fifth lumbar vertebra.

BONY PELVIS

The bones of the pelvic region consist of two hip bones (right and left), sacrum and coccyx. The right and left hip bones are joined anteriorly at the pubic symphysis and to the sacrum and coccyx posteriorly to form *pelvic girdle* or *bony pelvis* (Fig. 6.12). Above it

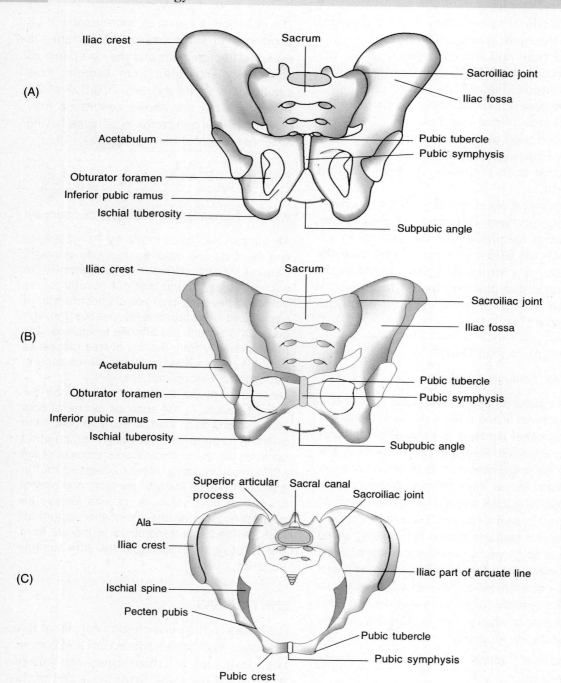

Fig. 6.12: The bony pelvis, (A) Male, (B) Female, (C) The female pelvis as seen from above. The inlet of female pelvis is large and oval in shape

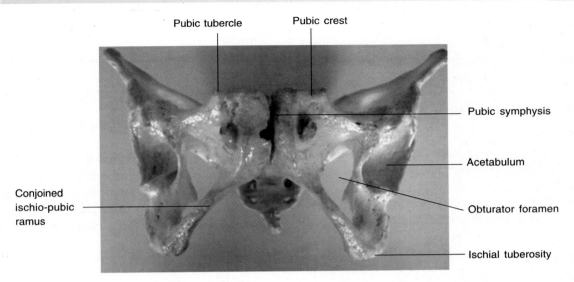

Pubic tubercle

Pubic crest

Pubic symphysis

Acetabulum

Obturator foramen

Ischial tuberosity

Conjoined ischio-pubic ramus

Fig. 6G: Anterior aspect of the female pelvis. Note the wide sub-pubic angle

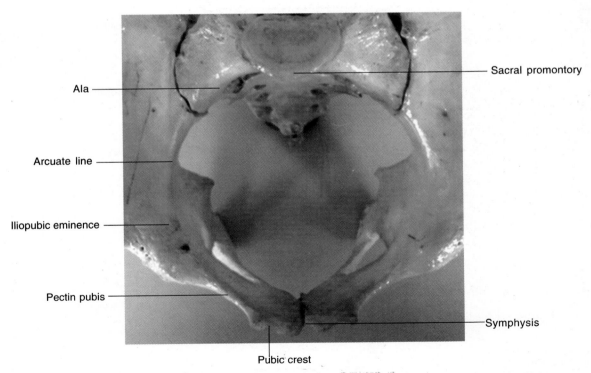

Sacral promontory

Ala

Arcuate line

Iliopubic eminence

Pectin pubis

Symphysis

Pubic crest

Fig. 6H: Superior aspect of the female pelvis. Note the shape and boundaries of pelvic inlet

articulates with the lumbar part of the vertebral column at the lumbosacral joint. Below it is attached to the lower limbs (femora) at hip joints.

Functions of the Bony Pelvis

- The bony pelvis is the basin shaped ring of bones, which protects the distal part of the intestine, urinary bladder and internal genital organs.
- The main function of the bony pelvis is to transmit the weight of the upper body from the vertebral column to the lower limbs.
- It transmits the thrust between vertebral column and lower limbs.
- Provides attachment to the powerful muscles.
- It gives passage to the fetus at the time of birth.

The bony pelvis is divided into *greater* and *lesser* pelvis (Figs. 6.13 and 6.14). The greater pelvis is also called as *false pelvis*. The lesser pelvis is called as *true pelvis*. The greater and lesser pelves are separated from each other

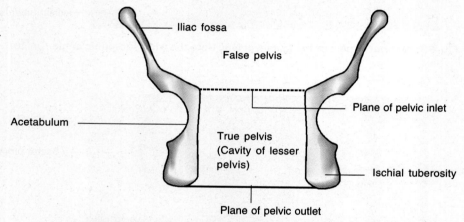

Fig. 6.13: Diagrammatic representation of the coronal section of pelvis

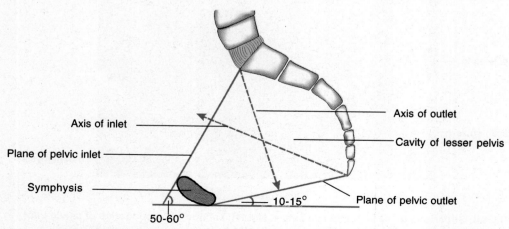

Fig. 6.14: Diagrammatic representation of the sagittal section of male pelvis

by an imaginary plane, i.e., *plane of pelvic inlet or pelvic brim).*

Greater Pelvis

The walls of the greater or false pelvis are formed by the iliac fossa of the hip bones and posteriorly by the ala of the sacrum. Anteriorly, the greater pelvis presents no bony wall.

Lesser Pelvis

The lesser or true pelvis presents an inlet (superior pelvic aperture), a pelvic cavity and an outlet (inferior pelvic aperture).

The Pelvic Inlet

The plane of pelvic inlet slopes obliquely downwards and forwards (Fig. 6.14). *The axis of the inlet* is determined by a line drawn perpendicular through the center of the plane. The plane of pelvic inlet makes an angle of 50 to 60 with the horizontal plane. The boundary of the pelvic inlet on each side is formed behind by the sacral promontory, anterior margin of the ala of the sacrum, the linea terminalis and the upper end of the symphysis pubis. (The linea terminalis of each hip bone consists of arcuate line of ilium,

iliopubic eminence, pectin pubis and pubic crest) (Fig. 6.12C).

The Cavity of the Lesser Pelvis

The cavity of the lesser pelvis extends downwards and backwards from the pelvic inlet and lies between inlet and outlet. Anteriorly, the cavity is bounded by the symphysis, body of the pubis and two rami of pubis. On each side, the wall is formed by ilium and ischium below the arcuate line. Posteriorly it is limited by the concave pelvic surface of the sacrum and coccyx. The posterior wall of the cavity is much longer than the anterior wall (Fig. 6.14).

The Outer or Inferior Pelvic Aperture (Pelvic Outlet)

It is bounded anteriorly by the lower margin of the symphysis pubis, anterolaterally by the conjoined ischiopubic rami, laterally by the ischial tuberosities, posterolaterally by sacrotuberous ligaments and posteriorly by the tip of the coccyx (Fig. 6.15). Thus the lower pelvic aperture is somewhat diamond shaped. The plane of pelvic outlet lies between lower border of symphysis pubis and the tip of coccyx. A line drawn perpendicular to the center of this plane is

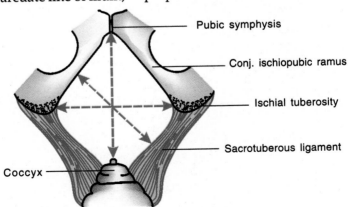

Pubic symphysis

Conj. ischiopubic ramus

Ischial tuberosity

Sacrotuberous ligament

Coccyx

Fig. 6.15: Various diameters of pelvic outlet

known axis of pelvic outlet (Fig. 6.14). The plane of pelvic outlet makes an angle of 10 to 15 with the horizontal plane.

The Axis of Pelvic Cavity

The axis of the pelvic cavity is an imaginary axis passing through the pelvic cavity between inlet and outlet of the pelvic cavity (Fig. 6.16). This axis is concave anteriorly and passes parallel to the sacrococcygeal curve.

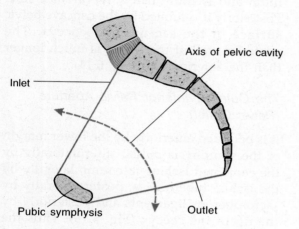

Fig. 6.16: The axis of the pelvic cavity

The axis of the pelvic cavity is important because through this axis passes the head of the fetus during childbirth. Hence, the axis of the pelvic cavity is also called as axis of birth canal.

Diameters of the Pelvis

The diameter of pelvic inlet and outlet are important in females due to child bearing.

Measurements of the Inlet in Adult Females

Anteroposterior diameter: It extends between the middle of sacral promontory to the upper margin of symphysis pubis. It measures about 105 to 110 mm (Fig. 6.17).

The transverse diameter: It is the widest measurement across the inlet. It measures about 125 to 130 mm.

The oblique diameter: It is measured from the sacroiliac joint of one side to iliopubic eminence of other side. It measures about 120 to 125 mm.

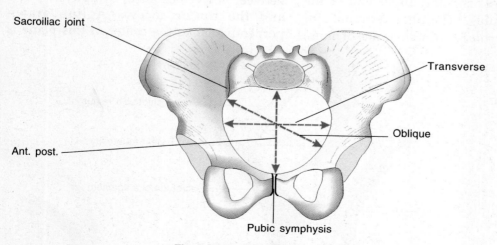

Fig. 6.17: Various diameters of inlet of pelvis

Table 6.1: Differences between male and female pelves		
Features	*Male pelvis*	*Female pelvis*
General features	Male pelvis is thick and heavy. Muscular impressions are more prominent.	Female pelvis is thin and muscular impressions are less prominent.
Acetabulum	The acetabulum is large for transmission of greater body weight as compared to females. The distance between pubic symphysis to the anterior margin of the acetabulum is less as compared to the diameter of the acetabulum.	The acetabular cavity is small. The distance between pubic symphysis to the anterior margin of the acetabulum is more as compared to the transverse diameter of the acetabulum.
Greater sciatic notch	The angle of greater sciatic notch is narrow. Its depth is less.	The angle of the greater sciatic notch is wide. Its depth is more.
Base of sacrum	For transmission of greater body weight in the males, the width of the body of the sacrum is more than the width of the ala.	The width of the body of the sacrum is less than the width of ala.
Sub-pubic angle	The sub-pubic angle is narrow. It is between 50 to 60 degrees (Fig. 6.18).	The sub-pubic angle is wide, about 90 degrees (Fig. 6.18).
Obturator foramen	Because of the narrow sub-pubic angle the obturator foramen is round or ovoid.	Because of the wide sub-pubic angle it is triangular in shape.
Chilotic line	The chilotic line extends from the ilio pubic eminence to the anterior margin of the auricular surface and thence to the iliac crest. In males the anterior portion of the chilotic line is shorter than posterior segment.	In females, the anterior portion of the chilotic line is longer than the posterior segment.
The pelvic inlet	It is heart shaped and all distances are smaller than females.	It is rounded in shape and all diameters are longer than males.
Cavity of lesser pelvis	Cavity is narrow and deep (long) so that there is less space in the true pelvis.	Cavity is wide and shallow so that there is more space in the true pelvis.
The pelvic outlet	Comparatively small.	Comparatively large because it has to accommodate the passage of fetal head at birth.
Ischiopubic index of Washburn	$\dfrac{\text{The length of pubis} \times 100}{\text{Height of ischium}}$ It is less than 90.	$\dfrac{\text{The length of pubis} \times 100}{\text{Height of ischium}}$ It is more than 90.
Index of "height of pelvic cavity/length of arcuate line" of Pal (2009)	The index of height of pelvic cavity (distance between iliopubic eminence to the ischial tuberosity) and the length of arcuate line is a very useful guide. In the male the index is usually above 78.	In females this index is below 78.

Measurements of the Outlets in Adult Females

The anteroposterior diameter: It is measured from the lower border of symphysis pubis to the tip of the coccyx. It is about 125 mm.

The transverse diameter: It is the distance between two ischial tuberosities. It measures about 110 to 118 mm.

The oblique diameter: It is the distance between the junction of ischiopubic ramus of one side and the midpoint of the sacrotuberous ligament of the opposite side.

Anatomical Position of the Pelvis

Hold the articulated pelvis in such a way that the upper end of the pubic symphysis and the anterior superior iliac spines lie in the same vertical plane (place these points against a wall).

• In this position the tip of the coccyx lie almost at the level of upper margin of symphysis pubis.
• The pelvic inlet faces forwards and upwards and the pelvic outlet faces downwards and backwards.
• In this position sacrum faces downwards and forwards.

Differences Between Male and Female Pelves

The pelves of males and females differ significantly. These differences are due to childbearing function in females. For identification of sex from human skeletal remains, the pelvis or even a single hip bone is the most useful because here the sexual differences are clearly defined (Table 6.1).

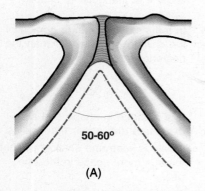

(A)

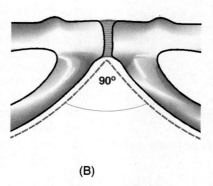

(B)

Fig. 6.18: The sub-pubic angle in (A) Male is 50 to 60° and in (B) Female about 90°

Further Readings

• Pal G.P. and Routal R.V. (1987). *Journal of Anatomy* (U.K.) 152, 93-105.

• Pal G.P. (1989). *Journal of Anatomy* (U.K.) 162, 9-17.
• Pal G.P., Choudhary S and Bose S (2009). *The Journal of ASI* 58(2), 173-178.

7) *Bones of the Head and Neck Regions*

The bones of the head and neck regions consist of skull, cervical vertebrae and hyoid bone.

- The skull forms the skeleton of the head region. The skull contains a large cavity for the lodgment of the brain (called as cranial cavity) and two small cavities for the lodgment of the eyes (called as orbits). On the anterior aspect of the skull there are two openings, i.e., opening of nasal cavity and the opening of the oral cavity (mouth).
- Below the skull the skeleton of the neck is formed by the seven cervical vertebrae.
- The hyoid bone is a small bone, present in the upper part of neck in front of the 3rd cervical vertebra.

SKULL

The skull (the skeleton of head) is formed by 22 bones. These bones are firmly joined to one another and are immobile except the bone of the lower jaw (mandible), which moves at temporomandibular joint. The skull is divided into two parts, i.e., *cranium* and *facial skeleton.*

Cranium

- It is also known as *neuro-cranium, brain box or calvaria.* The cranium is upper and posterior part of the skull (Fig. 7.1). Cranium means skull minus the mandible.
- It consists of 8 bones. Out of these 8 bones 4 are unpaired (*frontal, occipital, sphenoid*

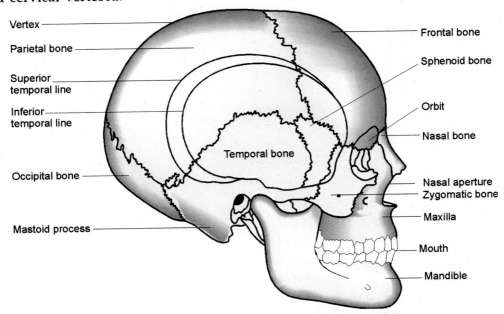

Vertex

Parietal bone

Superior temporal line

Inferior temporal line

Occipital bone

Mastoid process

Frontal bone

Sphenoid bone

Orbit

Nasal bone

Temporal bone

Nasal aperture
Zygomatic bone

Maxilla

Mouth

Mandible

Fig. 7.1: Skull as seen in lateral view (norma lateralis)

and *ethmoid*) and 2 are paired (*parietal and temporal*).

- The joints between these bones are immobile and are known as *sutures*.
- The cranium has a dome like roof (called as *vault or skull cap*) and a floor or cranial base (called as *basi-cranium,* Fig. 7.2).

Facial Skeleton (Viscerocranium)

- Facial skeleton forms the anterior part of the skull (Fig. 7.3). It contains orbital and nasal cavities and includes upper and lower jaws (maxillae and mandible).
- In addition to frontal bone, facial skeleton consists of 14 bones. Out of these 6 are paired (*lacrimal, nasal, maxillae, zygomatic, palatine and inferior nasal conchae*). While, mandible and *vomer* are single bones.

Anatomical Position of the Skull

To obtain the anatomical position of the skull, it is kept in the *"Frankfurt horizontal plane"*.
- Hold the skull in such a way that the inferior border of the orbit and superior border of external acoustic meatus of right and left sides lie in the same horizontal plane (Fig. 7.1).

Table 7.1: Bones forming the skull		
	Paired	Unpaired
Cranium	Parietal bones Temporal bones	Frontal bone Occipital bone Sphenoid bone Ethmoid bone
Facial skeleton	Maxillae Zygomatic bones Nasal bones Lacrimal bones Palatine bones Inferior conchae	Mandible Vomer bone Frontal bone

Students are suggested to identify various bones of a dry skull with the help of Figs. 7.1 to 7.7. Once they are able to identify various bones in skull then only they should proceed to study the details of skull as seen from various aspects. A dry skull may be viewed from:

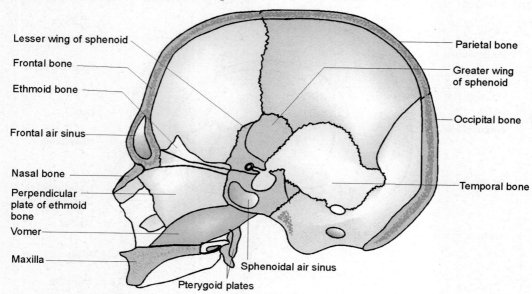

Lesser wing of sphenoid
Frontal bone
Ethmoid bone
Frontal air sinus
Nasal bone
Perpendicular plate of ethmoid bone
Vomer
Maxilla
Pterygoid plates
Sphenoidal air sinus
Parietal bone
Greater wing of sphenoid
Occipital bone
Temporal bone

Fig. 7.2: Sagittal section of the skull showing cranial and nasal cavities

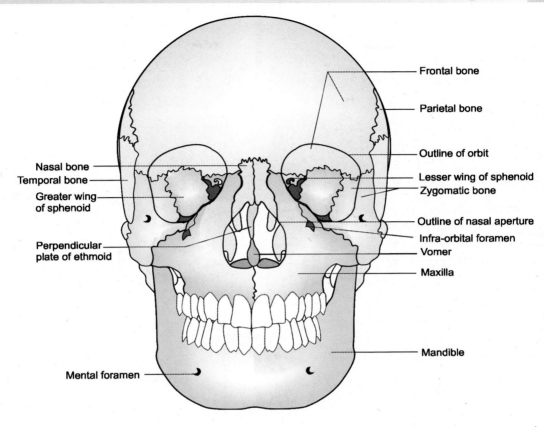

Fig. 7.3: Skull as seen from anterior (frontal) aspect (norma frontalis)

- Above (*norma verticalis*, Fig. 7.4).
- Behind (*norma occipitalis*, Fig. 7.5).
- Front (*norma frontalis*). The walls of the *orbital cavity* may also be examined from this view (Fig. 7.3).
- And from the side (*norma lateralis*, Fig. 7.1).
- Below (*norma basalis externa*, Fig. 7.6).
- The roof of the calvaria (*skull cap*, Fig. 7.4) may be removed by a transverse cut to examine the inside of the floor of the cranium. The interior of the base of the skull (*norma basalis interna*) is divided into three cranial fossae, i.e., anterior, middle and posterior (Fig. 7.7). The inner aspect of the skull cap is shown in Fig. 7.8.

- The section of the skull in para-median plane will help us to study the *nasal cavity* (Fig. 7.2).

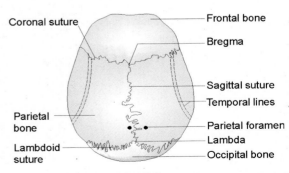

Fig. 7.4: Skull as seen from above (norma verticalis)

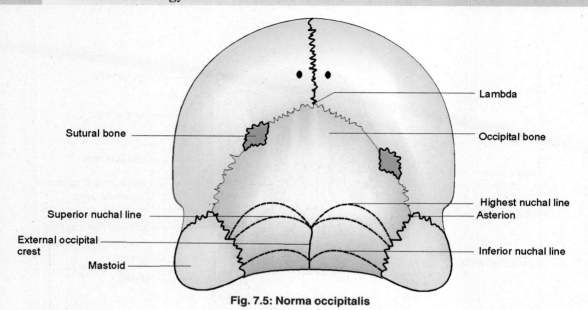

Fig. 7.5: Norma occipitalis

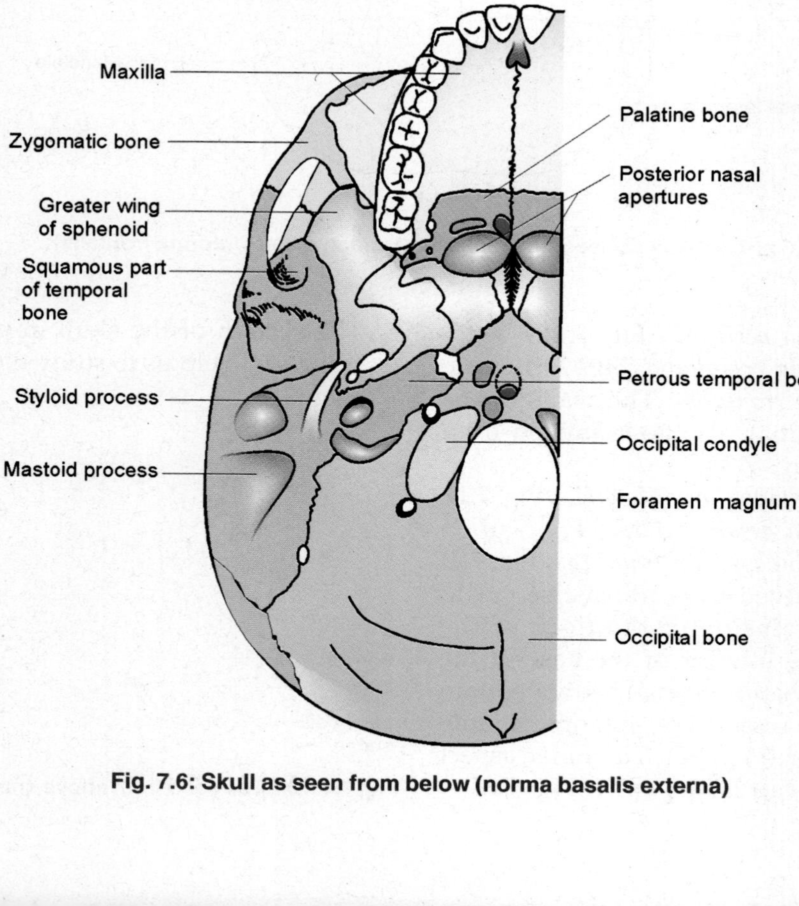

Fig. 7.6: Skull as seen from below (norma basalis externa)

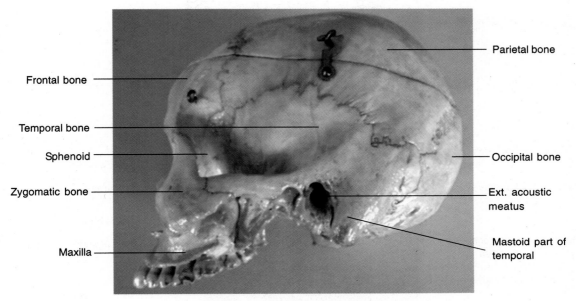

Fig. 7A: Norma lateralis (minus mandible)

Frontal bone
Temporal bone
Sphenoid
Zygomatic bone
Maxilla

Parietal bone
Occipital bone
Ext. acoustic meatus
Mastoid part of temporal

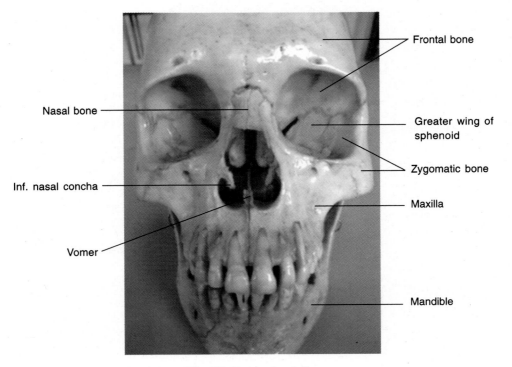

Nasal bone
Inf. nasal concha
Vomer

Frontal bone
Greater wing of sphenoid
Zygomatic bone
Maxilla
Mandible

Fig. 7B: Norma frontalis

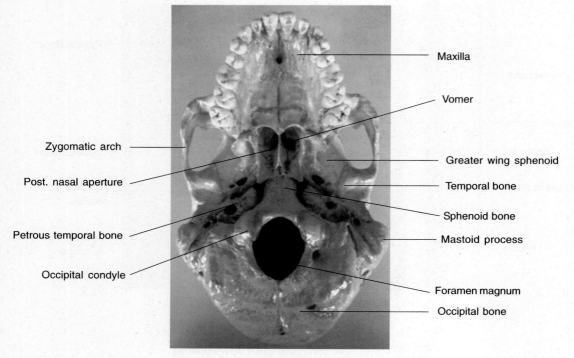

Fig. 7C: Norma basalis externa

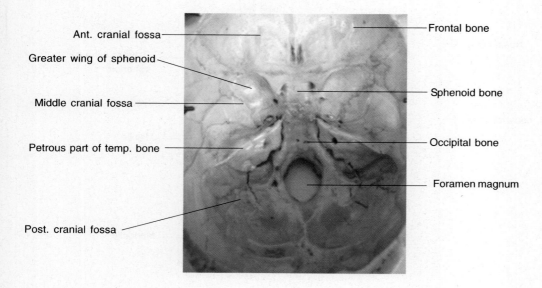

Fig. 7D: Norma basalis interna

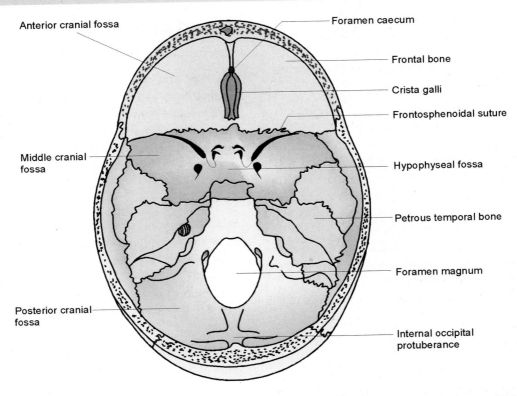

Anterior cranial fossa

Foramen caecum

Frontal bone

Crista galli

Frontosphenoidal suture

Middle cranial fossa

Hypophyseal fossa

Petrous temporal bone

Foramen magnum

Posterior cranial fossa

Internal occipital protuberance

Fig. 7.7: The base of skull as seen from internal aspect (norma basalis interna) showing anterior, middle and posterior cranial fossae

SUPERIOR ASPECT OF THE SKULL (NORMA VERTICALIS)

When the skull is viewed from above it appears oval in shape (Figs. 7.4 and 7.8). It is relatively wider nearer its occipital pole (posteriorly). The bones forming the skull-cap (roof of the brain box) are visible from this aspect.

Bones Forming the Norma Verticalis

- *Frontal bone*—It is a single bone that forms the anterior part of the norma verticalis.
- *Parietal bones* —These are paired bones and lie posterior to the frontal bone on each side of the midline.

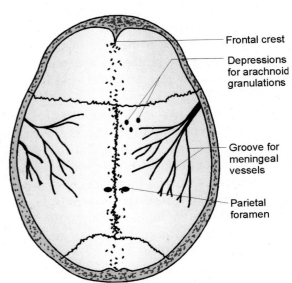

Frontal crest

Depressions for arachnoid granulations

Groove for meningeal vessels

Parietal foramen

Fig. 7.8: The inner aspect of skull cap

- *Occipital bone*—It is a single bone and lies posterior to the parietal bones.

Sutures (Joints) Present in the Norma Verticalis

Following three sutures and their meeting points are seen in this norma:

- *Coronal suture*—It lies between frontal and right and left parietal bones.
- *Sagittal suture*—It is present in midline between right and left parietal bones.
- *Lambdoid suture*—It lies between occipital and two parietal bones.
- *Bregma*—It is a landmark point, where coronal and sagittal sutures meet each other. It is present in midline.
- *Lambda*—It is present at the junction of the sagittal and lambdoid sutures.

Features of Norma Verticalis

- The *parietal foramen* is present near the sagittal suture about 3.5 cm anterior to the lambda. It transmits a small emissary vein, which connects the superior sagittal sinus with the veins of scalp.
- *Parietal eminence* is the area of the maximum convexity on the parietal bone. It is present on the posterolateral aspect of the parietal bone.
- *Superior and inferior temporal lines* are seen on the lateral side of frontal and parietal bones. The superior temporal line gives attachment to the *epicranial aponeurosis* and *temporal fascia*. The inferior temporal line gives attachment to the *temporalis muscle*.
- *The vertex* is the highest point of the skull and is situated near the mid point of the sagittal suture (Fig. 7.1).

APPLIED IMPORTANCE

Metopic Suture

The right and left halves of the frontal bone is ossified from separate centers. There exists a *frontal suture* between two frontal bones before the age of 6 years. In some adult skull this suture may persist in full or in part and is known as *metopic suture* (Fig. 7.9).

Sutural Bones

Isolated small bony ossicles (bones) are sometimes observed along the lambdoid and sagittal sutures. These are called as *sutural bones* (Fig. 7.5). They are formed due to ossification from separate centers.

Fontanelle

In the skull of newborn there are membranous gaps at the site of bregma and lambda. These are called *anterior* and *posterior fontanelles* respectively (Fig. 7.10). The anterior fontanelle closes (membranous gap of anterior fontanelle is replaced by bone) by 18 months of age, while posterior closes by 2 to 3 months of age. Following are the functions of fontanelle:

- Fontanelle allows moulding of skull during birth, as the head passes through the birth canal.
- They also allow the brain to grow.
- An increased intracranial tension leads to the bulging of the anterior fontanelle.
- Similarly, depression of anterior fontanelle indicates dehydration.
- One can easily draw the blood for testing or inject drugs in the superior sagittal sinus through anterior fontanelle.

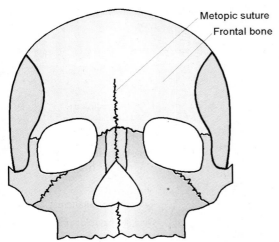

Fig. 7.9: The presence of partial metopic suture

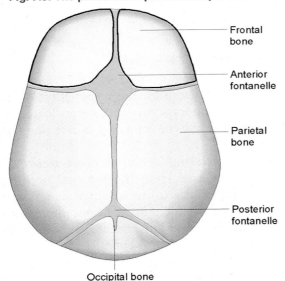

Fig. 7.10: Superior view of newborn skull showing fontanelle

FURTHER DETAILS

Sutural Bones

Sutural bones (wormian bones) are small irregular shaped ossicles, often found within the cranial sutures and at the fontanelles, especially in relation to parietal bone. The number of sutural bones is usually limited to

---

two or three, but they may be present in great number in skulls of hydrocephalics. The mechanism responsible for formation of sutural bones is not precisely known. Some believe that these are formed due to increased head stress (due to pathology and hydrocephaly) while others are of the opinion that sutural bones are derived from normal developmental process and are genetically determined. A study by Pal *et al.* (1986a) compared the cranial capacity in skull with and without sutural bones and observed no significant difference. This was interpreted as indicating that sutural bones are not formed secondary to stress. In another study (Pal *et al.*, 1986b) they observed no significant difference in occurrence of sutural bones in three different morphological forms of skull (dolichocephalic, mesocephalic and brachyce-phalic). This finding was also interpreted as indicating that sutural bones are not formed secondary to stress but are genetically determined.

Pal *et al.* (1986a) have also used the incidence of sutural bones as anthropological marker to measure the distance of one group of population from another.

THE POSTERIOR ASPECT OF THE SKULL (NORMA OCCIPITALIS)

Bones Seen in Norma Occipitalis (Refer Fig. 7.11)

- Right and left parietal bones.
- Squamous part of the occipital bone.
- Mastoid part of right and left temporal bone.

Sutures (Joints) Seen in Norma Occipitalis

- Posterior part of the sagittal suture in midline.

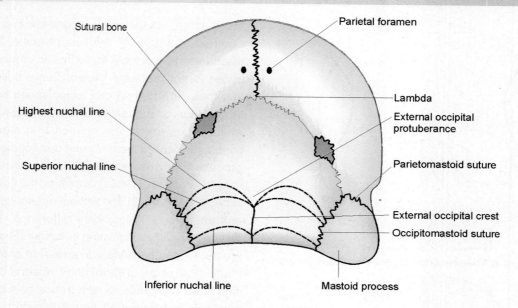

Fig. 7.11: Skull as seen from behind (norma occipitalis)

- Lambdoid suture between two parietal and occipital bone.
- Right and left parietomastoid sutures between parietal and the mastoid part of the temporal bones.
- Right and left occipitomastoid sutures between occipital and mastoid bones.
- The parietal, occipital and mastoid bones, on each side, meet at a point, which is known as *asterion*. It is at a junction of the lambdoid, parietomastoid and occipito-mastoid sutures.

Features

- The *external occipital protuberance* is a palpable midline elevation. The highest point on this protuberance is also known as *inion*.
- The *superior nuchal lines* extend laterally from each side of the external occipital protuberance to the mastoid process.

These lines mark the upper limit of the neck. The trapezius and sternocleidomas-toid muscles are attached to this line (Fig. 7.26).

- The *external occipital crest* descends downwards from the external occipital protuberance to the foramen magnum. It gives attachment to the *ligamentum nuchae*.
- The right and left *inferior nuchal lines* run laterally from the crest.
- The right and left *highest nuchal* lines are present just above the superior nuchal lines. These lines give attachment to the epicranial aponeurosis and to the occipital belly of the occipitofrontalis (Fig. 7.26).
- The *mastoid foramen* is situated close to the occipitomastoid suture and transmits an emissary vein and meningeal branch of occipital artery.
- One or more *sutural bones* may be present at the lambda, lambdoid suture or at asterion (Fig. 7.11).

- Between superior and inferior nuchal lines *semispinalis capitis* and *obliquus capitis superior* muscles are attached.
- Between inferior nuchal line and posterior margin of the foramen magnum *rectus capitis posterior major and minor* are attached.

ANTERIOR ASPECT OF THE SKULL (NORMA FRONTALIS)

This aspect of the skull forms the facial skeleton and consists of forehead, orbits, nasal region, malar prominence and upper and lower jaws (Figs. 7.3 and 7.12).

Bones Seen in the Norma Frontalis

Identify the following bones from above downwards:

- Frontal bone.
- Nasal bones.
- Zygomatic bones.
- Maxillae.
- Mandible.

The frontal bone and mandible are single bones, while nasal, zygomatic and maxillae are paired bones.

Sutures (Joints) Seen in the Norma Frontalis

Identify the following sutures, which are present close to the median plane:

- The *fronto-nasal suture* is present between nasal process of the frontal bone and nasal bones.

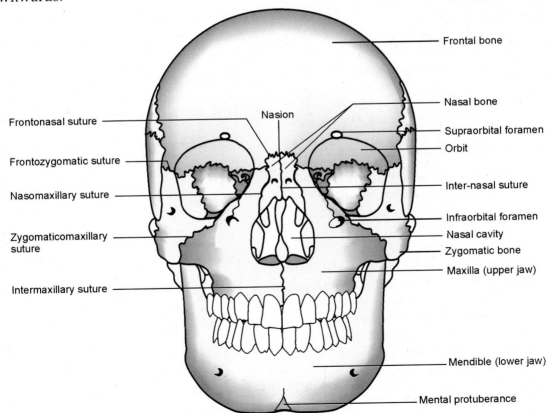

Fig. 7.12: Features of norma frontalis

- The *fronto-maxillary suture* is present between the nasal part of the frontal bone and the frontal process of maxilla.
- The inter-nasal suture is present in midline between two nasal bones above the nasal aperture.
- The *naso-maxillary suture* is present between lateral border of nasal bone and the frontal process of the maxilla.
- The *inter-maxillary suture* is present between right and left maxilla below nasal aperture.

Identify the following sutures present laterally in the norma frontalis:

- The *fronto-zygomatic suture* is present between zygomatic process of the frontal bone and the frontal process of zygomatic bone. This suture is present on the lateral border of the orbit.
- The *zygomatico-maxillary suture* is between zygomatic process of maxilla and the maxillary process of the zygomatic bone.
- The *nasion* is the meeting point of inter-nasal and fronto-nasal sutures. It is present in midline at the root of the nose.

Features of the Norma Frontalis

For the ease of understanding norma frontalis is studied under the following headings:

Forehead

The squamous part of the frontal bone forms the skeleton of the forehead. In the fetal and infant skulls the two halves of the frontal bone are separated by the *frontal suture*. Two frontal bones remain separated upto 6 years of age. In some adults this suture may persist as *metopic* suture (Fig. 7.9).

- The *glabella* is the smooth, slightly depressed middle area just above the nasion.

- The superciliary arches are curved elevations above the medial part of supra-orbital margins. They extend laterally from glabella.
- The *frontal eminences* are paired rounded elevations above the superciliary arches.

Orbital Openings

Each orbital opening is quadrangular in shape and presents four margins (Fig. 7.13).

- The *supraorbital margin* is formed by frontal bone. This border presents a supraorbital notch or foramen at the junction of medial 1/3 with lateral 2/3. The supraorbital nerve and vessels pass to the forehead through the supraorbital notch or foramen. The supratrochlear vessels and nerve pass medial to the supraorbital notch.
- The *infraorbital margin* is formed by the maxilla medially and zygomatic bone laterally. The infraorbital foramen is present just below this margin, which transmits infraorbital nerve and vessels.

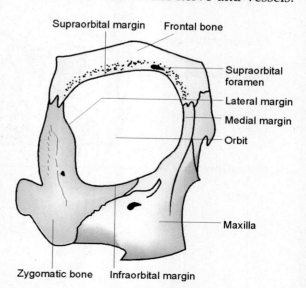

Fig. 7.13: The orbital opening

- The *lateral margin* of the orbit is formed by the zygomatic and frontal bones.
- The *medial margin* is formed by the frontal bone and the frontal process of the maxilla. The detail description of the orbital cavity is given later.

Malar Prominence

The prominence of the cheek is formed by the zygomatic bone. It is situated infero-lateral to the orbit. The zygomatico-facial foramen is present on the bone, which transmits the nerve of the same name.

Anterior Nasal Aperture

The nasal aperture is piriform in shape (Fig. 7.14).
- It is bounded above by the right and left nasal bones, while lateral and inferior boundaries are formed by the nasal notches of right and left maxilla.
- The anterior nasal spine is a median bony projection from the maxillae.
- Margins of the anterior nasal aperture give attachment to the nasal cartilage.
- In the depth of anterior nasal aperture nasal septum can be seen in midline. This septum separates the cavity of nose into right and left nasal cavities. A detail description of nasal cavity is given later in this chapter.

Upper Jaw (Maxillae)

The upper jaw is formed by the right and left maxilla (Figs. 7.3 and 7.12).
- The *alveolar process* of maxilla bears the sockets for the upper teeth.
- The root of canine tooth produces an elevation on the upper jaw, which is known as *canine eminence.*
- The *canine fossa* is situated just lateral to the canine eminence.
- The *incisive fossa* is situated above the incisor teeth.

Lower Jaw (Mandible)

The lower jaw is formed by the mandible. The mandible is the only movable bone of the skull.
- The alveolar processes house the lower teeth.
- The *mental foramen* is present below the 2nd premolar teeth. It gives passage to the mental nerve and vessels.
- The anterior surface of the symphysis menti presents a triangular elevation, the *mental protuberance* (Fig. 7.12).

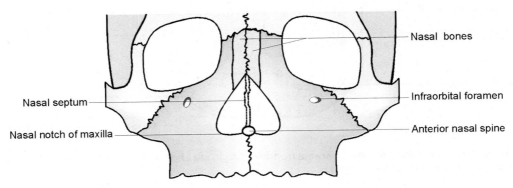

Fig. 7.14: Figure showing the margins of anterior nasal aperture

The mandible is described in more detail in Chapter 8.

Attachment of Muscles in the Norma Frontalis

Students should study the attachment of muscles on norma frontalis with the help of Fig. 7.15.

THE ORBITAL CAVITY

We have already studied the orbital margins in this chapter. Here, we shall study the walls and various openings of the orbital cavity (Fig. 7.16).

The orbit is like a four-sided pyramid. It has a base, an apex, roof, floor, medial wall and lateral wall.

The Base

The base of the orbit is the orbital opening. It has four margins, i.e., upper, lateral, medial and inferior margins (Fig. 7.13).

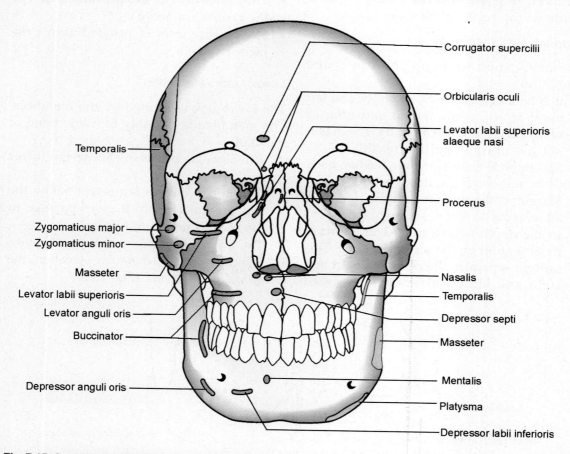

Fig. 7.15: Attachment of the muscles on norma frontalis. Origin are shown on the right side (in brick red color) and insertion on left side (in blue color)

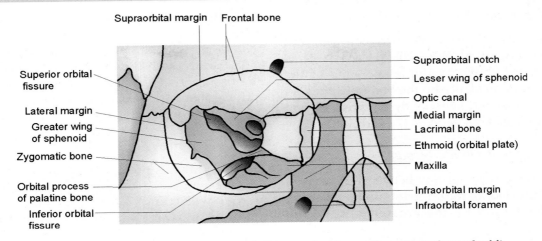

Fig. 7.16: The orbital cavity. Schematic diagram showing walls and openings of orbit

The Apex

The apex of the orbit lies posteriorly.

The Medial Wall

The medial wall of the orbit, from anterior to posterior, is formed by the frontal process of the maxilla, lacrimal bone, orbital plate of the ethmoid and body of the sphenoid.

- Most anteriorly the medial wall shows a deep groove called as lacrimal groove. This groove lodges the lacrimal sac. It is bounded anteriorly and posteriorly by the anterior and posterior lacrimal crests, respectively.
- Most of the medial wall is formed by the orbital plate of the ethmoid.
- The anterior and posterior ethmoidal foramina are present at the superior border of this bone.

The Superior Wall or Roof

The superior wall is formed mainly by the orbital plate of the frontal bone. Most posteriorly, a small part of the roof is also formed by the lesser wing of the sphenoid.

- Anteromedially there is presence of a small depression called as the *trochlear fossa*, which gives attachment to the pulley for superior oblique muscle.
- Anterolaterally there is a deep fossa called as *lacrimal fossa* for lacrimal gland.

The Lateral Wall

It is formed anteriorly by zygomatic bone and posteriorly by the greater wing of the sphenoid.

The Inferior Wall or Floor

It is mainly formed by the maxilla. The small anterolateral part of the floor is also formed by the zygomatic bone. Most posteriorly the floor is formed by the orbital process of the palatine bone (Fig. 7.18).

Fissures, Canals and Foramina of the Orbital Cavity

The orbital cavity communicates with the neighbouring regions of the skull through superior and inferior orbital fissures, optic and infraorbital canals and various foramina.

The Superior Orbital Fissure

It is present posteriorly between roof and lateral wall of the orbital cavity. It is bounded above by the lesser wing of the sphenoid, medially by the body of sphenoid and below and laterally by the greater wing of the sphenoid (Figs. 7.17 and 7.18).

The Inferior Orbital Fissure

It is present posteriorly between lateral wall and the floor of the orbit. It is bounded above and laterally by the greater wing of the sphenoid and below and medially by the maxilla (Fig. 7.18). It communicates posteriorly with the pterygopalatine fossa and laterally with the infratemporal fossa. The fissure gives passage to the maxillary and zygomatic nerves, emissary veins and infraorbital vessels.

The Optic Canal

The optic canal is present at the apex of the orbital cavity at the junction of the roof and medial wall (Fig. 7.18). It is bounded medially by the body of sphenoid and

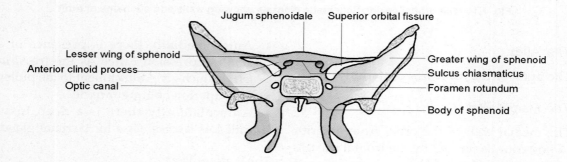

Fig. 7.17: Schematic diagram showing superior orbital fissure as seen from posterior aspect of sphenoid bone

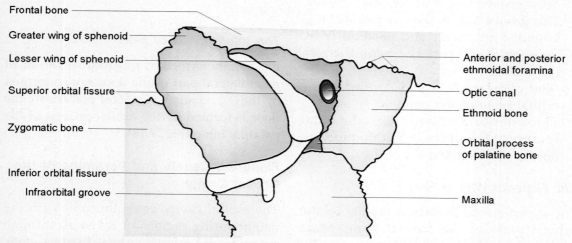

Fig. 7.18: Schematic diagram of a part of right orbit showing boundaries of superior and inferior orbital fissures

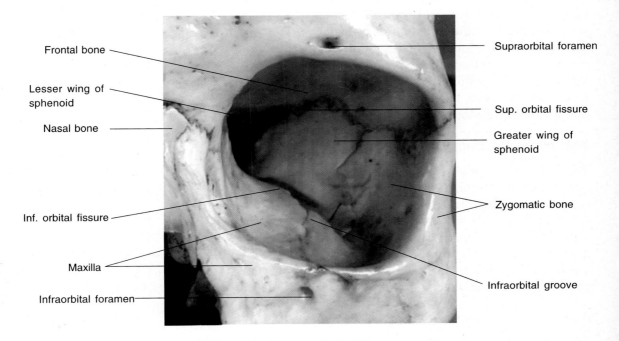

Fig. 7E: Orbital margin and orbital cavity

Frontal bone

Lesser wing of sphenoid

Nasal bone

Inf. orbital fissure

Maxilla

Infraorbital foramen

Supraorbital foramen

Sup. orbital fissure

Greater wing of sphenoid

Zygomatic bone

Infraorbital groove

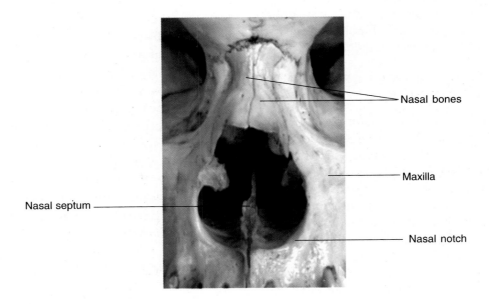

Fig. 7F: The margin of anterior nasal aperture

Nasal bones

Maxilla

Nasal notch

Nasal septum

laterally by lesser wing. It communicates with the middle cranial fossa and transmits the optic nerve along with its meningeal covering and ophthalmic artery. A common tendinous ring, which gives origin to four recti muscles of eye, is attached surrounding the opening of the optic canal.

The Infraorbital Canal

The infraorbital canal is present in the bony substance of the maxilla. The canal is continuous posteriorly on the floor of the orbit as infraorbital groove and opens anteriorly at the infraorbital foramen. It gives passage to the infraorbital nerve and vessels. The infraorbital nerve is the continuation of maxillary nerve.

Anterior and Posterior Ethmoidal Foramina

These two small foramina are present at the upper border of the orbital plate of ethmoid (at the junction of roof and medial wall of orbit, Fig. 7.18). These foramina transmit the anterior and posterior ethmoidal nerves and vessels to the anterior cranial fossa.

THE LATERAL ASPECT OF THE SKULL (NORMA LATERALIS)

This aspect of the skull is formed by cranial and facial bones. The posterosuperior region of norma lateralis (cranial part) includes temporal fossa, external acoustic meatus and mastoid part of the temporal bone. The anteroinferior part of the norma lateralis (facial part) includes zygomatic arch, infratemporal fossa, lateral aspect of the maxilla and mandible.

Bones Seen in the Norma Lateralis

Identify the following bones on the lateral aspect of the skull:

- *Frontal.*
- *Parietal.*
- *Occipital.*
- *Nasal.*
- *Maxilla.*
- *Zygomatic.*
- *Sphenoid.*
- *Temporal.*
- *Mandible.*

Sutures (Joints) of the Norma Lateralis

Many sutures, which are seen on this aspect, have been already observed while studying norma frontalis, verticalis and occipitalis. Hence, we shall study the sutures present in the central region of the norma lateralis (Fig. 7.19).

H Shaped Suture

The H shaped suture is the meeting point of four bones, i.e., frontal, parietal, greater wing of sphenoid and squamous part of the temporal bone. A small circular area enclosing parts of all four bones is called as *"pterion"*. The pterion lies on the floor of the temporal fossa. The horizontal limb of the suture is the joint between anteroinferior angle of the parietal bone and the greater wing of the sphenoid (*parietosphenoid suture*). The greater wing of the sphenoid articulates anteriorly with the frontal bone (at *frontosphenoidal suture*) and posteriorly with the squamous part of the temporal bone (at *temporosphenoidal suture*) (Fig. 7.19).

The Parietosquamous and Parietomastoid Sutures

The lower border of the parietal bone articulates anteriorly with the squamous part of temporal bone at *parietosquamous suture* and posteriorly with the mastoid bone at *parieto-mastoid suture.*

Lambdoid Suture

At this suture the posterior border of the parietal bone articulates with the occipital bone (Fig. 7.19).

Occipitomastoid Suture

Here the occipital bone articulates with the mastoid part of the temporal bone.

Features of the Norma Lateralis

Following bony features are seen on the lateral aspect of the skull (Fig. 7.19):

Temporal Lines

Superior and inferior temporal lines are seen on this aspect (Fig. 7.1). The superior line starts at the zygomatic process of frontal bone. It arches upwards and backwards crossing the coronal suture and fades away on the temporal bone. It gives attachment to epicranial aponeurosis and temporal fascia.

The inferior line starts along with the superior and runs inferior and parallel to it. Posteriorly, it runs downwards and forwards on the temporal bone to become continuous with the supramastoid crest. The crest is further continuous anteriorly with the posterior root of the zygoma. The inferior temporal line limits the attachment of temporalis muscle.

Zygomatic Arch

The zygomatic arch is formed by the articulation between the temporal process of zygomatic and the zygomatic process of temporal bone. At the posterior end and at its lower border, the zygomatic arch bears a

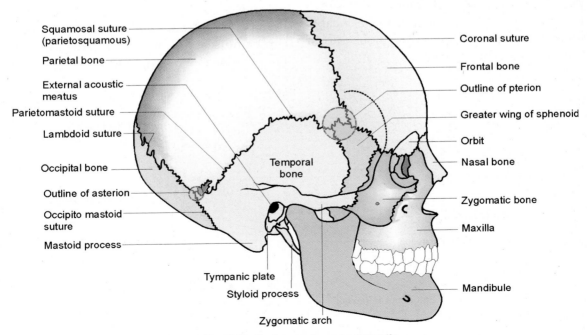

Fig. 7.19: Features of norma lateralis

tubercle called as *root of zygoma*. Here the zygomatic arch divides into anterior and posterior roots. Trace the posterior root backwards along the lateral margin of the mandibular fossa, and then above the external acoustic meatus to become continuous with the *supramastoid crest*. The anterior root passes horizontally as articular tubercle, which lies anterior to the mandibular fossa.

The temporal fascia is attached to the upper border of the zygomatic arch. The lower border and inner surface of the arch gives origin to the masseter muscle.

The External Acoustic Meatus

The tympanic plate and squamous part of the temporal bone form the external acoustic meatus. The roof and upper part of the posterior wall is formed by squamous temporal bone, while lower part of the posterior wall, floor and anterior wall by the tympanic plate. The margin of the meatus gives attachment to the cartilaginous part of the external acoustic meatus.

Suprameatal Triangle

It is a depression, situated postero-superior to the external acoustic meatus (Fig. 7.20). It is bounded above by the supramastoid crest, in front by the posterosuperior margin of the external acoustic meatus and behind by a vertical line drawn along the posterior margin of the meatus. Deep to this triangle lies the mastoid antrum.

Mastoid Process

The mastoid part of the temporal bone lies behind the external acoustic meatus. It is continuous above with the squamous temporal bone. The mastoid process is downward conical projection from the mastoid part of the temporal bone. The asterion is the junctional point of three sutures, i.e., parietomastoid, occipitomastoid and lambdoid (Fig. 7.19).

The external surface of the mastoid provides attachmnent to the sternocleidomastoid, splenius capitis and longissimus capitis muscles. A mastoid foramen pierces the bone near the occipitomastoid suture. It

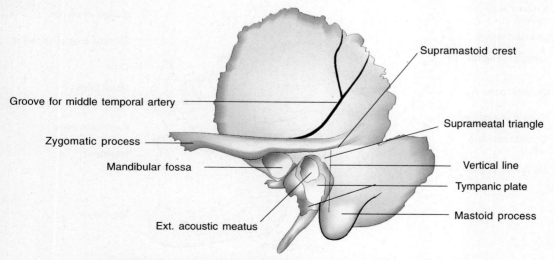

Fig. 7.20: The suprameatal triangle and the features of surrounding area

Groove for middle temporal artery

Zygomatic process

Mandibular fossa

Ext. acoustic meatus

Supramastoid crest

Suprameatal triangle

Vertical line

Tympanic plate

Mastoid process

transmits an emissary vein from the sigmoid sinus and the meningeal branch of occipital artery.

The Styloid Process

The styloid process is seen when skull is viewed from the lateral side. It is about 2 to 5 cm long process projecting downwards, forwards and medially (Fig. 7.21). It is situated in front of the mastoid process on a deeper plane. It gives attachment to the styloglossus, stylohyoid and stylopharyngeus muscles. The stylohyoid and stylomandibular ligaments are also attached to it (Fig. 7.31).

Temporal Fossa

This is a shallow fossa that lies above the zygomatic arch. The temporalis muscle is located in this fossa. This fossa is bounded:

- Posteriorly and superiorly by temporal lines.
- Anteriorly by the temporal surface of the frontal and zygomatic bones.
- Inferiorly by the superior border of the zygomatic arch and supramastoid crest (on the lateral side). Inferiorly on the medial side by the infratemporal crest of the greater wing of the sphenoid. Between zygomatic arch and infratemporal crest temporal fossa communicates below with the infratemporal fossa.
- Floor of the temporal fossa is formed by the part of the frontal, parietal, temporal and greater wing of the sphenoid bones. The circular area enclosing all these four bones and H shaped suture is called as *pterion* (Fig. 7.19). It is situated 4 cm above the mid point of the zygomatic arch and 3.5 cm behind the frontozygomatic suture. The middle meningeal vein, anterior branch of middle meningeal artery and

stem of the lateral sulcus of brain lie deep to the pterion.

The *contents* of the temporal fossa are temporalis muscle, deep temporal vessels and nerves and zygomaticotemporal nerve.

Infratemporal Fossa

It is an irregular fossa below the zygomatic arch and behind the maxilla. It communicates above with the temporal fossa deep to zygomatic arch (Figs. 7.21 and 7.22).

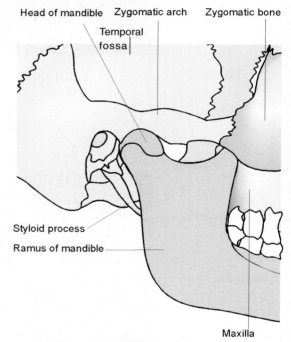

Fig. 7.21: Lateral wall of infratemporal fossa

Boundaries

- *Anterior wall:* The posterior surface of the body of maxilla bone. The surface of the maxilla shows many perforations (openings) for posterosuperior alveolar nerves and vessels (Fig. 7.22).
- *Medial wall:* It is formed by the lateral pterygoid plate and pyramidal process of palatine bone. The junction of anterior and

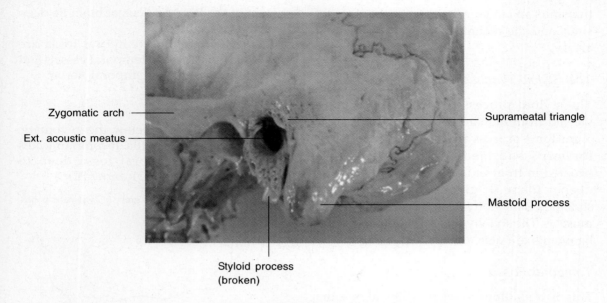

Zygomatic arch

Ext. acoustic meatus

Suprameatal triangle

Mastoid process

Styloid process
(broken)

Fig. 7G: Suprameatal triangle

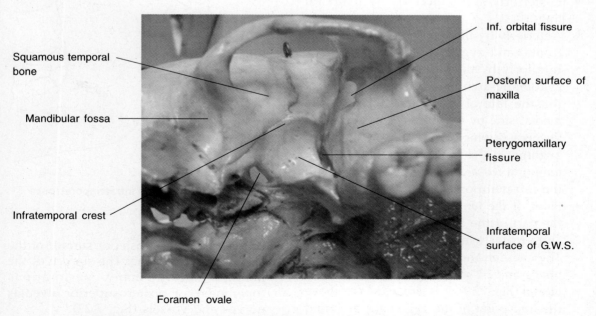

Inf. orbital fissure

Squamous temporal
bone

Posterior surface of
maxilla

Mandibular fossa

Pterygomaxillary
fissure

Infratemporal crest

Infratemporal
surface of G.W.S.

Foramen ovale

Fig. 7H: Infratemporal fossa, roof and anterior wall, as seen from inferior aspect

medial wall shows a fissure called as *pterygomaxillary fissure.* Deep to the fissure lies the *pterygopalatine fossa* (Fig. 7.22).

- *Lateral wall:* It is formed by ramus and coronoid process of the mandible (Fig. 7.21).
- *Roof:* The roof is formed by the infra-temporal surface of the greater wing of sphenoid. At the junction of roof and anterior wall, lies the lateral part of inferior orbital fissure through which infratemporal fossa communicates with the orbit (Fig. 7.22). Foramen ovale and foramen spinosum are present in the roof of the infratemporal fossa.
- *Floor:* It is not bounded but open.
- *Posterior wall:* It is also open.

The *contents* of the infratemporal fossa are as mentioned below:

- Lateral and medial pterygoid muscles and lower part of the temporalis.
- The maxillary artery and its branches, pterygoid venous plexus.
- Mandibular, maxillary and chorda tympani nerve and otic ganglion.

Pterygopalatine Fossa

It is a small pyramidal space situated below the apex of the orbit and deep to the pterygomaxillary fissure.

Boundaries

- *Anterior:* Posterior surface of the body of the maxilla.
- *Posterior:* Root of the pterygoid process and the anterior surface of greater wing of the sphenoid.
- *Medial:* The perpendicular plate of the palatine bone.
- *Lateral:* It is open and communicates with infratemporal fossa through pterygo-maxillary fissure. *(The pterygomaxillary fissure (Fig. 7.22) is a triangular gap bounded anteriorly by maxilla and posteriorly by pterygoid process. It transmits the third part of the maxillary artery, maxillary nerve and posterior superior alveolar nerve and vessels).*
- *Roof:* Medially it is bounded by the body of the sphenoid and orbital process of the

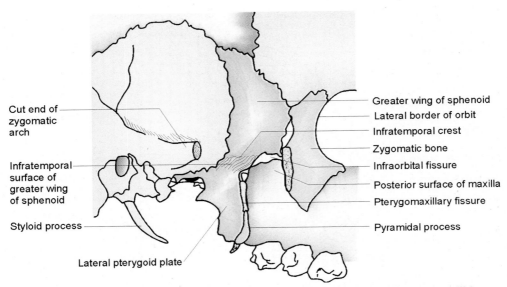

Cut end of zygomatic arch

Infratemporal surface of greater wing of sphenoid

Styloid process

Lateral pterygoid plate

Greater wing of sphenoid
Lateral border of orbit
Infratemporal crest
Zygomatic bone
Infraorbital fissure
Posterior surface of maxilla
Pterygomaxillary fissure
Pyramidal process

Fig. 7.22: Infratemporal fossa seen after removal of zygomatic arch and mandible (showing anterior and medial wall)

palatine bone. Laterally it communicates with the inferior orbital fissure.

- *Floor:* It is closed due to the fusion of anterior and posterior wall.

Communications of the Pterygopalatine Fossa

It communicates with the following:

- *The orbit*–Through the infraorbital fissure.
- *The infratemporal fossa*–Through pterygomaxillary fissure.
- *The nasal cavity*–Through sphenopalatine foramen.
- *The middle cranial fossa*–Through the foramen rotundum.
- *The foramen lacerum*–Through pterygoid canal.

Contents of the Pterygopalatine Fossa

- Maxillary nerve, pterygopalatine ganglion and its branches.

- The third part of the maxillary artery.

THE NORMA BASALIS EXTERNA

To visualize the base of the skull, it is necessary to detach the mandible from the rest of the skull. The base of the skull is formed, from anterior to posterior, by maxillae, palatine, vomer, sphenoid, temporal and occipital bones (Fig. 7.6). For the convenience of description, the norma basalis is divided into anterior, middle and posterior parts by two imaginary horizontal lines. The first imaginary horizontal line is drawn along the posterior border of the hard palate and second line passes through the anterior margin of the foramen magnum.

Anterior Part of the Norma Basalis Externa

It is formed by the *alveolar arch* of maxilla and *hard palate* (Fig. 7.23).

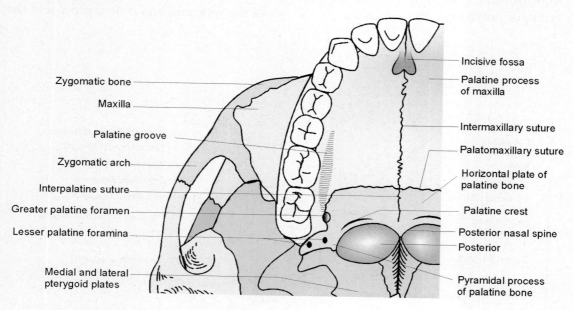

Fig. 7.23: The anterior part of norma basalis externa. Some parts of middle portion are also shown

Alveolar Arch

Alveolar arch is formed by the alveolar processes of right and left maxillae. It is horseshoe shaped and possesses the sockets for the roots of the teeth of upper jaw.

Hard Palate

- The hard palate lies within the alveolar arch.
- The anterior 2/3 of the hard palate is formed by the palatine processes of right and left maxillae (Fig. 7.23).
- The posterior 1/3 is formed by the horizontal plates of palatine bones.

Features

Sutures (joints) and foramina seen in the anterior part of the norma basalis.

Intermaxillary, interpalatine and palato-maxillary sutures are shown in Fig. 7.23. All the above three sutures are collectively called as *cruciform suture*.

The Greater Palatine Foramen

It is situated just medial to third molar, posterior to the palatomaxillary suture. A groove runs forward from this foramen. This foramen transmits *greater palatine vessels and nerves.*

The Lesser Palatine Foramina

These are two to three small foramina situated behind the greater palatine foramen. These foramina are present in the pyramidal process of the palatine bone. The *lesser palatine vessels and nerves* pass through these foramina.

The Incisive Fossa

It is a triangular depression in the median plane behind the central incisor teeth. The right and left lateral walls of the fossa bear lateral incisive foramen, which communicate with the floor of the nasal cavity. It gives passage to the *nasopalatine nerve* and *greater palatine vessels.*

Pyramidal Process of the Palatine Bone

It occupies the gap between the lower end of medial and lateral pterygoid plates.

The Posterior Nasal Spine

It is a midline projection from the posterior border of the hard palate. It gives attachment to the *musculus uvulae* on each side.

Palatine Crest

It is a curved ridge a little in front of the posterior border of hard palate. It gives attachment to the *palatine aponeurosis* and the tendon of *tensor veli palatini.*

Premaxilla

It is a triangular piece of maxilla holding four incisor teeth. In young persons a suture may be seen running from the posterior part of the incisive fossa laterally between the lateral incisor and canine teeth, separating the premaxilla from the rest of the maxilla.

The Middle Part of the Norma Basalis Externa (Fig. 7.24)

The middle part extends between two imaginary lines, i.e., the anterior line drawn along the posterior border of hard palate and posterior line drawn along the anterior margin of foramen magnum. The structures present in the region are divided into median area and right and left areas.

The bones present in the median area, from anterior to posterior are:

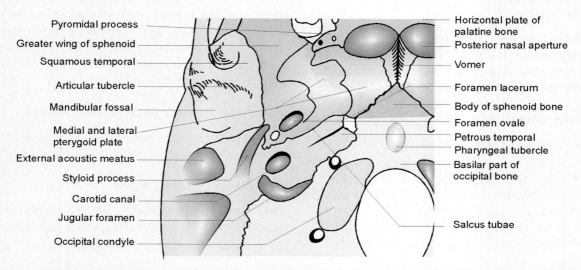

Pyramidal process
Greater wing of sphenoid
Squamous temporal
Articular tubercle
Mandibular fossal
Medial and lateral pterygoid plate
External acoustic meatus
Styloid process
Carotid canal
Jugular foramen
Occipital condyle

Horizontal plate of palatine bone
Posterior nasal aperture
Vomer
Foramen lacerum
Body of sphenoid bone
Foramen ovale
Petrous temporal
Pharyngeal tubercle
Basilar part of occipital bone
Salcus tubae

Fig. 7.24: The middle part of norma basalis externa. Some part of anterior and posterior portions of norma basalis are also shown

- Posterior border of vomer.
- Body of sphenoid.
- Basilar part of the occipital bone.

The bones in the lateral area are:

- Medial and lateral pterygoid plates on the right and left side. These plates are the part of the sphenoid bone.
- Infratemporal surface of greater wing of sphenoid. It is situated lateral to the pterygoid plates.
- Temporal bone with its squamous, tympanic and petrous parts.

Features

A. The Posterior Nasal Apertures and Related Structures

These are quadrilateral in shape and situated above the posterior margin of the hard palate.

- The posterior border of vomer separates the right and left apertures from each other, thus forms the *medial boundary* of each aperture.

- The superior surface of the horizontal plate of palatine bone forms the *floor* of the posterior nasal aperture.
- *Laterally*, each aperture is bounded by the perpendicular plate of palatine bone, which articulates with the medial pterygoid plate, posteriorly.
- The *roof* of the aperture is formed by the ala of the vomer and the sphenoidal process of the palatine bone.

The upper border of the vomer splits into two alae close to the inferior surface of the body of sphenoid (Fig. 7.25). The midline groove between two alae of the vomer articulates with the sphenoidal rostrum (which is a midline ridge on the inferior surface of the body of sphenoid). The under surface of the ala of the vomer, on each side, is overlapped by the vaginal process, which arises from the root of the medial pterygoid plate. There exists a narrow vomerovaginal canal between the undersurface of the ala of vomer and upper surface of vaginal process.

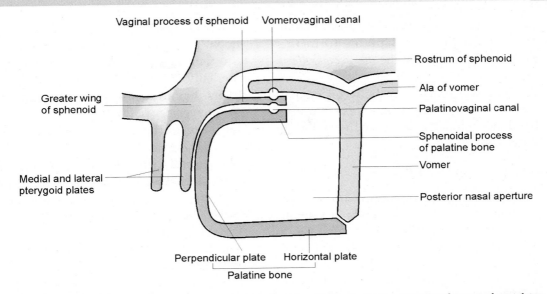

Fig. 7.25: Schematic diagram showing the bones forming the boundaries of posterior nasal aperture

It is present occasionally and gives passage to the pharyngeal vessels and nerve. From the upper end of the perpendicular plate of palatine bone there extends a sphenoidal process medially, which overlaps the undersurface of vaginal process. A narrow canal is present between the undersurface of the vaginal process and superior surface of the sphenoidal process. It is called as palatinovaginal canal and gives passage to the pharyngeal vessels and nerve. The vomerovaginal canal is situated posteriorly as compared to the palatinovaginal canal.

B. The Median Bar of Bone

Just behind the alae of vomer bone there is the presence of broad bar of bone in the midline. It extends upto the foramen magnum. It is formed by two bones, i.e., under surface of the body of sphenoid and basilar part of the occipital bone (Fig. 7.24). These two bones (body of sphenoid and occipital bone) remain separated from each other by a cartilaginous synchondrosis joint which later fuses at about the 25 years of age.

A median elevation is seen just in front of foramen magnum. It is known as the pharyngeal tubercle, which gives attachment to *pharyngeal raphae* and fibers of *superior constrictor*. Note the attachment of *longus capitis* and *rectus capitis* anterior on the basilar part of the occipital bone (Fig. 7.26).

C. Pterygoid Processes

Each pterygoid process descends vertically downwards from the junction of the body and greater wing of sphenoid.

- The anterior surface of the root of pterygoid process forms the posterior wall of *pterygopalatine fossa*.
- The pterygoid process consists of medial and lateral *pterygoid plates*.
- The pterygoid plates unite anteriorly and enclose a fossa (*pterygoid fossa*), which faces posterolaterally.

- The anterior surface of the fused medial and lateral pterygoid plates form the posterior boundary of the *pterygomaxillary fissure.*
- At the lower end, a gap between medial and lateral pterygoid plates is occupied by the *pyramidal process* of the palatine bone (Fig. 7.24).

The Medial Pterygoid Plate

- Trace above the posterior border of medial pterygoid plate. It ends in a small fossa the *"scaphoid fossa"*. It gives attachment to the *tensor veli palatini* (Fig. 7.26).
- The lower end of its posterior border projects downwards and laterally as a hook, the *hamulus.* Around the hamulus the tendon of tensor veli palatini turns medially to enter the soft palate. The hook of the hamulus also gives attachment to *the pterygomandibular raphe.*
- Its posterior border gives attachment to the *pharyngobasilar fascia.*
- An angular process (*process tubarius*) projects backwards from the middle of the posterior border of medial pterygoid plate. This process supports the medial end of auditory tube.
- The lower end of the posterior border with pterygoid hamulus gives origin to the superior constrictor muscle.

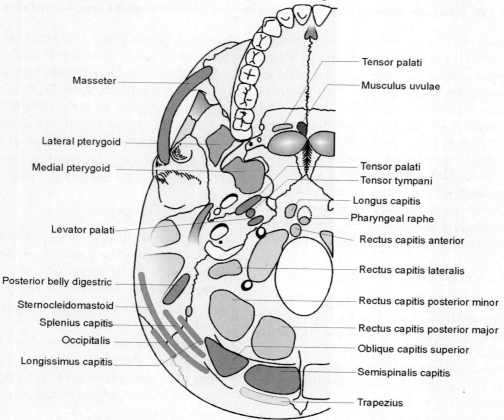

Fig. 7.26: Attachment of muscles on norma basalis externa

The Lateral Pterygoid Plate

- The medial surface of the lateral pterygoid plate gives origin to the deep head of medial pterygoid muscle (Fig. 7.26).
- Its lateral surface gives origin to lower head of lateral pterygoid muscle.

D. Infratemporal Surface of the Greater Wing of Sphenoid

This surface of the greater wing of sphenoid extends laterally from the root of the lateral pterygoid plate. It is pentagonal in shape and forms the roof of the infratemporal fossa (Fig. 7.27).

- Anteriorly it forms the posterolateral border of the inferior orbital fissure.
- Laterally the surface is limited upto the infratemporal crest. Beyond this crest the greater wing extends in the temporal surface.
- Postero-laterally it articulates with the squamous part of the temporal bone (Fig. 7.24).
- Posteromedially it articulates with the

petrous part of the temporal bone. At the junction of these two bones a sulcus is formed, which is known as *sulcus tubae*. *The sulcus lodges the cartilaginous part of the auditory tube.*

- The posterior most part of this bone projects down as the spine of the sphenoid.

The spine of the sphenoid gives attachment to:

Ligaments–Sphenomandibular, pterygospinous and anterior ligament of the malleus.

Muscles–Posterior fibres of tensor veli palatine.

Related structures – Auriculotemporal nerve (laterally) chorda tympani nerve and auditory tube (medially).

- The infratemporal surface of the greater wing of sphenoid gives origin to the upper head of lateral pterygoid muscle.
- This surface presents two foramina, i.e., foramen ovale and spinosum. The foramen ovale is oval in shape and present posterolateral to the root of the lateral pterygoid plate. Foramen spinosum is

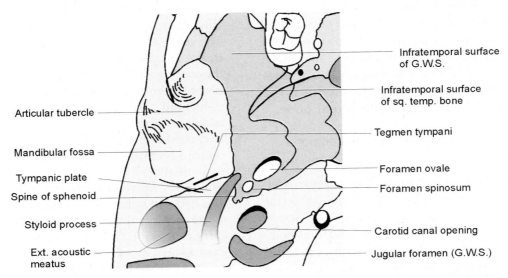

Fig. 7.27: The infratemporal surface of the greater wing of sphenoid (G.W.S.) and squamous temporal bone

small rounded foramen situated postero-lateral to foramen ovale. It is present anteriomedial to the spine of the sphenoid. Sometimes a small foramen may be seen medial to the foramen ovale, *emissary sphenoidal foramen.*

E. The Infratemporal Surface of the Squamous Part of the Temporal Bone

This part is present posterolateral to the greater wing of the sphenoid and along with the infratemporal surface of the greater wing of sphenoid it also forms the roof of the infratemporal fossa.

- When zygomatic process is traced backwards this surface presents a tubercle (tubercle of the root of zygoma) where zygomatic process divides into anterior and posterior roots.
- The anterior root runs medially anterior to the mandibular fossa and bears an *articular tubercle* (Fig. 7.27).
- The posterior root forms the lateral boundary of the mandibular fossa. Behind the articular tubercle the mandibular fossa is deep depression.
- Both the articular tubercle and mandibular fossa, are articular in nature and articulates with the head of the mandible.
- The posterior part of the mandibular fossa is non-articular and formed by the tympanic plate of the temporal bone.

F. The Tympanic Part of the Temporal Bone

The tympanic plate forms the anterior wall, floor and lower most part of the posterior wall of external acoustic meatus.

- The squamous part of the temporal bone and tympanic plate unite with each other at *squamotympanic fissure,* which is present in the floor of the mandibular fossa.

- The *tegmen tympani* part of the petrous temporal bone may project in the medial part of the squamotympanic fissure (Fig. 7.27).
- The presence of the tegmen tympani divides the squamotympanic fissure into a *petrosquamous fissure* and a *petrotympanic fissure.*
- The petro-tympanic fissure gives passage to chorda tympani nerve, anterior tympanic artery and anterior ligament of malleus.

G. The Inferior Surface of Petrous Part of Temporal Bone

The petrous part of the temporal bone is situated behind the greater wing of sphenoid and lateral to the body of sphenoid and basilar part of the occipital bone.

- The apex of the bone is separated from the body of sphenoid, root of pterygoid process and basilar part of the occipital bone by the foramen lacerum (Fig. 7.24).
- The carotid canal opens in the posterior wall of foramen lacerum, while the *pterygoid canal* opens into its anterior wall. The upper part of foramen lacerum is traversed by the internal carotid artery. The *nerve to the pterygoid canal* is formed in the foramen lacerum by the union of the *greater superficial petrosal* and *deep petrosal nerves.* The nerve then passes through pterygoid canal and enters the pterygo-palatine fossa.
- A quadrilateral area behind the apex of petrous bone gives origin to the *levator veli palatini* (Fig. 7.26).
- The lower opening of the carotid canal is situated just behind the quadrilateral area on the inferior surface of the petrous temporal bone. It transmits *the internal carotid* artery. Posterior to the lower opening of the carotid canal there lies the *jugular fossa.*

- The *sulcus tubae* is a groove, which lies between posteromedial margin of greater wing of sphenoid and the petrous part of the temporal bone (Fig. 7.24). It is occupied by the cartilaginous part of the *auditory tube.*

The Posterior Part of the Norma Basalis Externa

The posterior part lies behind the imaginary line drawn along the anterior margin of the foramen magnum. This part is also divided into median area and two lateral areas:

- The *median area* consists of foramen magnum and the squamous part of the occipital bone behind it. The condylar parts of the occipital bone are present on either side of the foramen magnum. The basilar part of the occipital bone lies anterior to the foramen magnum.
- The bones in the *lateral area,* on each side, are the mastoid and styloid process.

The Median Area

The foramen magnum is large and oval in shape. It connects the posterior cranial fossa above with the vertebral canal below.

The Basilar Part

The basilar part of the occipital bone is in direct continuity with the body of the sphenoid bone. These two bones are separated from each other by a primary cartilaginous joint in young but fuse with each other in adults. The pharyngeal tubercle is a small tubercle present on the inferior surface of the basilar part. It gives attachment to the pharyngeal raphe (Fig. 7.26).

The Foramen Magnum

The alar ligaments, which are attached on the lateral margins of the foramen magnum, divides the foramen into a small anterior and a large posterior parts. The structures passing through the anterior and posterior parts are shown in Fig. 7.29. The anterior and posterior margins of foramen magnum gives attachment to the anterior and posterior atlanto-occipital membranes respectively.

The Condylar Parts

The condylar parts of the occipital bone consist of right and left occipital condyles, which are situated on each side of the foramen magnum. The *jugular process* is present lateral to each condyle. The condyles are set obliquely and their inferior surface is convex and articular in nature. Each condyle articulates with the corresponding upper surface of the lateral mass of atlas vertebra (superior articular facet) to form atlanto-occipital joint.

There is the opening of hypoglossal or anterior condylar canal on the lateral border of the condyle near its anterior end (Fig. 7.28). It gives passage to the hypoglossal nerve, emissary vein and meningeal branch of ascending pharyngeal artery. A condylar fossa is present posterior to each condyle, which may show the presence of a canal (posterior condylar canal). It gives passage to the emissary vein which connects the sigmoid sinus to occipital veins.

The jugular process articulates laterally with the petrous temporal bone by a primary cartilaginous joint. The anterior margin of the jugular process is free and known as jugular notch. The jugular notch forms the posterior boundary of jugular foramen.

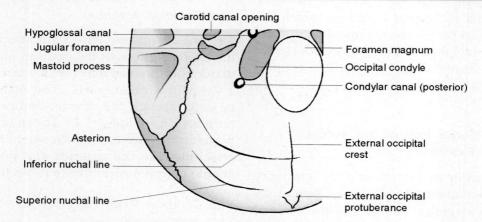

Fig. 7.28: The posterior part of the norma basalis externa

Carotid canal opening
Hypoglossal canal
Jugular foramen
Mastoid process
Asterion
Inferior nuchal line
Superior nuchal line
Foramen magnum
Occipital condyle
Condylar canal (posterior)
External occipital crest
External occipital protuberance

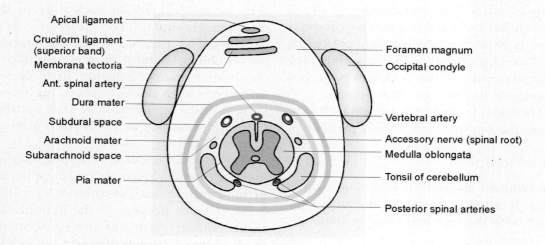

Fig. 7.29: Schematic diagram showing structure passing through foramen magnum

Apical ligament
Cruciform ligament (superior band)
Membrana tectoria
Ant. spinal artery
Dura mater
Subdural space
Arachnoid mater
Subarachnoid space
Pia mater
Foramen magnum
Occipital condyle
Vertebral artery
Accessory nerve (spinal root)
Medulla oblongata
Tonsil of cerebellum
Posterior spinal arteries

The Jugular Foramen

This irregular large foramen is bounded anteriorly by the posterior border of petrous temporal bone and posteriorly by the jugular notch of jugular process of occipital bone. It is divided into anterior, middle and posterior parts. The posterior part of the jugular foramen presents a jugular fossa, which is due to the presence of depression in the petrous temporal bone.

The mastoid canaliculi is an opening of a minute canal in the lateral wall of jugular fossa which transmits the auricular branch of vagus. The tympanic canaliculi is present on the ridge between jugular fossa and lower opening of the carotid canal. The structures passing through three divisions of the jugular foramen are shown in Fig. 7.30.

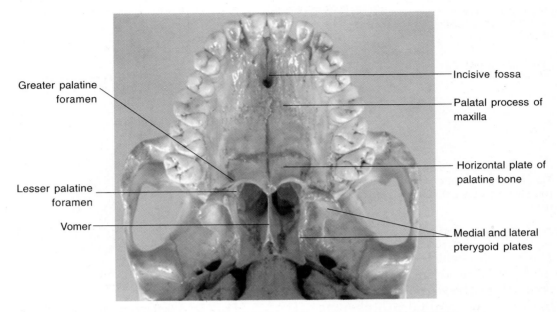

Greater palatine foramen

Lesser palatine foramen

Vomer

Incisive fossa

Palatal process of maxilla

Horizontal plate of palatine bone

Medial and lateral pterygoid plates

Fig. 7I: Anterior and part of middle portion of norma basalis externa

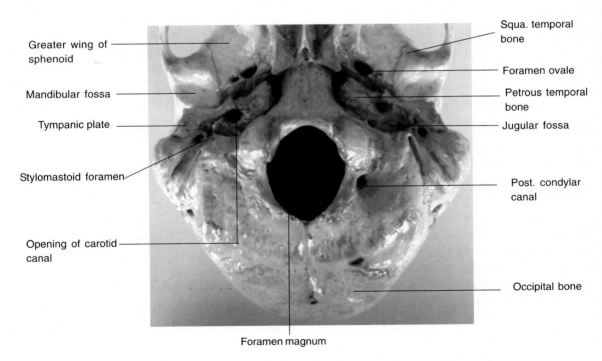

Greater wing of sphenoid

Mandibular fossa

Tympanic plate

Stylomastoid foramen

Opening of carotid canal

Squa. temporal bone

Foramen ovale

Petrous temporal bone

Jugular fossa

Post. condylar canal

Occipital bone

Foramen magnum

Fig. 7J: Part of middle and posterior part of norma basalis externa

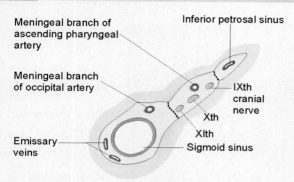

Meningeal branch of ascending pharyngeal artery

Inferior petrosal sinus

Meningeal branch of occipital artery

IXth cranial nerve

Xth

XIth

Emissary veins

Sigmoid sinus

Fig. 7.30: Schematic diagram showing structures passing through three divisions of left jugular foramen

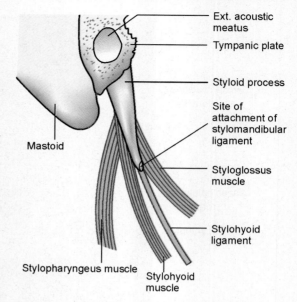

Ext. acoustic meatus

Tympanic plate

Styloid process

Site of attachment of stylomandibular ligament

Styloglossus muscle

Stylohyoid ligament

Mastoid

Stylopharyngeus muscle

Stylohyoid muscle

Fig. 7.31: Attachments of the styloid process

The Squamous Part

This part lies behind the foramen magnum. In the midline there extends an external occipital crest between foramen magnum and the external occipital protuberance. The upper end of the ligamentum nuchae is attached to the crest and protuberance. The superior and inferior nuchal lines and attachment of muscles in this area has already been described in "norma occipitalis". Students should refer Page 6 and Figs. 7.5 and 7.26

The Lateral Area

In the lateral area there are three important structures, i.e., styloid process, mastoid process and stylomastoid foramen.

Styloid Process

It is a long conical process, which projects downwards, forwards and medially below the tympanic part of the temporal bone.
• It lies lateral to the jugular fossa.
• It gives attachment to 3 muscles and two ligaments (Fig. 7.31).
• It is related laterally to the parotid gland and medially to the internal jugular vein.
• Near its base it is crossed by the facial nerve.

Mastoid Process

It is a conical projection from the mastoid part of the temporal bone. The mastoid process is situated posterolateral to the styloid process. A deep groove (*digastric groove*) is seen on its medial aspect, which gives attachment to the posterior belly of the digastric muscle.

Stylomastoid Foramen

The stylomastoid foramen is present between styloid and mastoid processes, i.e., posterolateral to the styloid process and anteromedial to the mastoid process. The stylomastoid artery and facial nerve pass through it.

THE INTERIOR OF THE SKULL

When the upper part of vault of the skull (skull cap or calvaria) is removed we may see the *inner surface of the cranial vault* and the *interior of the base of skull.*

Inner Surface of the Cranial Vault

The various bones and the intervening sutures forming the cranial vault are the same as observed in the norma verticalis.

- The *frontal crest* is the midline structure present most anteriorly (Figs. 7.7 and 7.32).

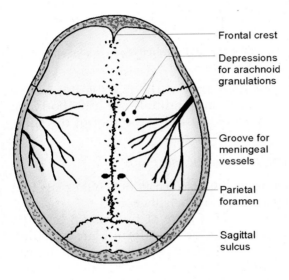

Fig. 7.32: The inner surface of cranial vault

Labels on figure:
- Frontal crest
- Depressions for arachnoid granulations
- Groove for meningeal vessels
- Parietal foramen
- Sagittal sulcus

- A groove extends anteroposteriorly in the median plane, from frontal crest to the internal occipital protuberance. This groove is known as *sagittal sulcus.*
- The *superior sagittal sinus* is lodged in the sagittal sulcus. At the internal occipital protuberance this sinus becomes continuous with the right transverse sinus.
- The frontal crest and the margins of the sagittal sulcus give attachment to the *falx cerebri.*
- Many small depressions (*granular pits*) are observed on each side of the sagittal sulcus. These are produced by the arachnoid granulations. Their number increases with the increasing age.

- Note the presence of parietal foramen on either side of sagittal suture about 3.5 cms anterior to lambda. These foramina transmit emissary vein.
- The inner aspect of the calvaria shows the presence of grooves for the meningeal vessels. These grooves run backwards and upwards from the anteroinferior angle of parietal bone.

Interior of the Base of the Skull

The internal aspect of the base of the skull (norma basalis interna) as seen after removal of the skull cap, can be divided into three fossae, i.e., *anterior, middle and posterior cranial fossae* (Fig. 7.7).

The Anterior Cranial Fossa

Bones of the Anterior Cranial Fossa

The anterior cranial fossa is formed by the frontal bone, cribriform plate of ethmoid, lesser wing of the sphenoid and the anterior part of the superior surface of body of the sphenoid (*jugum shpenoidale*).

Sutures of the Anterior Cranial Fossa

With the help of Fig. 7.33 identify fronto-ethmoidal, frontosphenoidal and spheno-ethmoidal sutures.

Borders

The anterior and lateral boundaries of the fossa are formed by the frontal bone. The posterior boundary is formed by the posterior border of the lesser wing of sphenoid, anterior clinoid process and the anterior border of sulcus chiasmaticus.

Floor

In the median region, the floor is formed by the cribriform plate of ethmoid and jugum

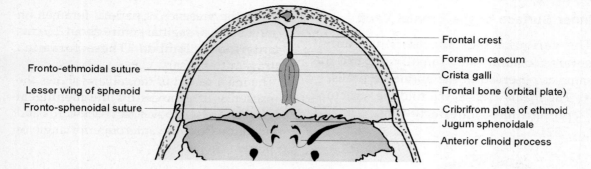

Fig. 7.33: The base of anterior cranial fossa. The adjacent part of middle cranial fossa is also shown

shpenoidale. While, the lateral region of the floor is formed by the orbital plates of frontal bone and the lesser wings of sphenoid, on each side.

Median Area of the Floor

- The most anterior structure in the mid line is the frontal crest.
- Posterior to the frontal crest a triangular process, the *crista galli*, is seen. It projects upwards from the cribriform plate and provides attachment to the falx cerebri.
- Between the frontal crest and crista galli identify the foramen caecum. Sometimes it transmits a vein from the nasal mucosa to the superior sagittal sinus.
- The cribriform plate of ethmoid is present on either side of crista galli between the orbital plates of frontal bone. The cribriform plate separates the anterior cranial fossa from the nasal cavity. It presents many small apertures through which pass the olfactory nerves from the nasal mucosa to the olfactory bulb.
- On each side of the cribriform plate there is the opening of anterior and posterior ethmoidal canals. Anterior canal transmits anterior ethmoidal vessels and nerve, while posterior canal transmits only posterior ethmoidal vessels.
- Posterior to the cribriform plate the

median area of the floor is formed by jugum sphenoidale of the body of sphenoid. It forms the roof of the sphenoidal air sinus.

Lateral Area of the Floor

On each side it consists of orbital plate and lesser wing of the sphenoid.

- The *orbital plate* of the frontal bone lie lateral to the cribriform plate on either side. It is convex and shows the impressions of cerebral gyri. Laterally it forms the roof of the orbit and medially the roof of the ethmoidal sinuses. Posteriorly, the orbital plates articulate with the anterior margin of the lesser wing of the sphenoid.
- The *lesser wings* of the sphenoid are continuous with the jugum sphenoidale medially. The posterior margin of the lesser wing is free and concave. It is related to the spheno-parietal sinus. The medial end of the posterior margin ends into anterior clinoid process, which gives attachment to free margin of tentorium cerebelli.

Middle Cranial Fossa

The middle cranial fossa is narrow in the middle and expanded laterally. It lodges hypophysis cerebri in middle and temporal lobes of the brain on each side.

Boundaries

- The *anterior boundary* of the middle cranial fossa separates the anterior and middle fossae from each other. It is formed by the posterior border of the lesser wing of sphenoid, anterior clinoid process and anterior border of sulcus chiasmaticus.
- The *posterior boundary* separates it from the posterior cranial fossa. It is formed by the superior border of petrous part of temporal bone, posterior clinoid process and dorsum sellae.
- On each side the middle cranial fossa is bounded by the greater wing of sphenoid, squamous part of temporal bone and parietal bone.

Floor of the Middle Cranial Fossa

It is shaped like a butterfly and consists of median and lateral parts (Fig. 7.34).

Median Part of the Floor of the Middle Cranial Fossa

- The median part is formed by the body of sphenoid. Most anteriorly *sulcus chiasmaticus* is present. It is a transverse groove, which becomes continuous laterally with the optic canal. The optic chiasma lies posterior to this groove.

- Each *optic canal* opens into orbit thus connects middle cranial fossa with orbit. It is bounded by anterior and posterior roots of lesser wing and body of sphenoid. This canal gives passage to the optic nerve, meninges and ophthalmic artery.
- Behind the sulcus chiasmaticus a saddle shaped depression is present on the superior surface of the body of sphenoid. It is known as *sella turcica*. The sella turcica consists of *tuberculum sellae, hypophyseal fossa* and *dorsum sellae* from anterior to posterior. The tuberculum sellae is median elevation just behind sulcus chiasmaticus. It receives the attachment of the anterior margin of diaphragma sellae. The hypophyseal fossa is a deep depression posterior to the tuberculum sellae. It lodges hypophysis cerebri. Deep to the hypophyseal fossa lies the sphenoidal air sinus.
- The *dorsum sellae* is a square like vertical plate of bone posterior to the hypophyseal fossa. The superior border of the dorsum sellae, on each side form the *posterior clinoid process* which give attachment to the attached margin of the tentorium cerebelli. While the superior border itself gives attachment to posterior margin of diaphragma sellae.

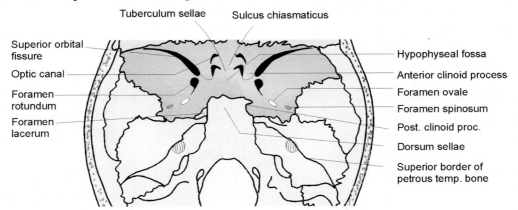

Fig. 7.34: The floor of middle cranial fossa. Adjacent part of anterior and posterior cranial fossae are also seen

- On each side of the body of sphenoid there is presence of a shallow groove called as carotid groove. This groove extends from the foramen lacerum to the medial side of anterior clinoid process. It lodges the internal carotid artery.

Lateral Part of the Floor of Middle Cranial Fossa

Laterally the floor of the middle cranial fossa is formed by three bones, i.e., cranial surface of the greater wing of sphenoid, squamous and petrous parts of the temporal bone (Fig. 7.34). Following fissures, foramina and grooves are observed in the floor of the fossa.

- *The superior orbital fissure* is a triangular oblique cleft present most anteriorly in the middle cranial fossa. It connects the middle fossa with the orbit. The fissure is bounded above by the lesser wing of sphenoid, below by greater wing and medially by the body of sphenoid. We have already seen (Page 12) that the fissure is divided into three parts by the attachment of a tendinous ring on the orbital surface of the fissure. The structures passing through three subdivisions of superior orbital fissure are shown in Fig. 7.35.

- The *foramen rotundum* is situated in the greater wing of sphenoid just inferomedial to the medial end of the superior orbital fissure. It opens anteriorly into the pterygopalatine fossa and transmits the maxillary nerve.

- The *foramen ovale* is situated in the greater wing of sphenoid posterolateral to the foramen rotundum. It opens into the infratemporal fossa and transmits the mandibular nerve.

- The *foramen spinosum* is also present in the greater wing of sphenoid, posterolateral to the foramen ovale and communicates with the infratemporal fossa. It gives passage to the middle meningeal artery and other structures.

- Sometimes the *emissary sphenoidal* foramen is present between foramen rotundum and foramen ovale. It transmits emissary vein. Similarly, sometimes a foramen is present between foramen ovale and spinosum, which transmits lesser petrosal nerve. It is called as *foramen innominatum.*

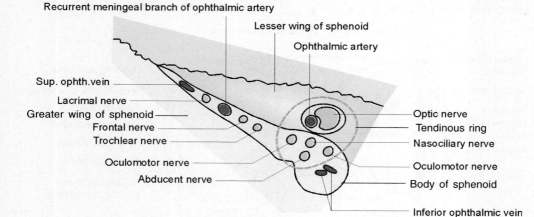

Fig. 7.35: Structures passing through right superior orbital fissure

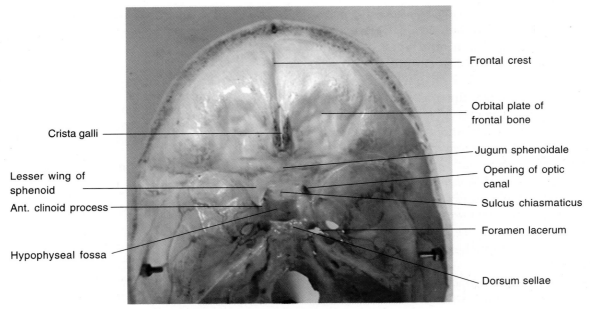

Frontal crest

Orbital plate of frontal bone

Crista galli

Jugum sphenoidale

Opening of optic canal

Lesser wing of sphenoid

Ant. clinoid process

Sulcus chiasmaticus

Foramen lacerum

Hypophyseal fossa

Dorsum sellae

Fig. 7K: Anterior and middle part of the norma basalis interna

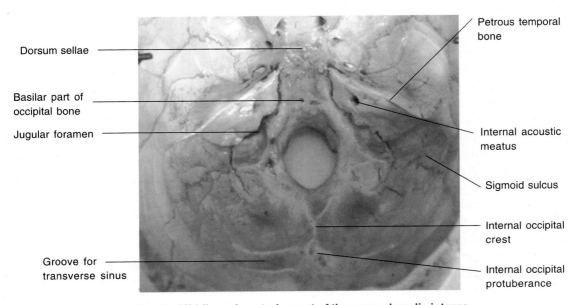

Petrous temporal bone

Dorsum sellae

Basilar part of occipital bone

Jugular foramen

Internal acoustic meatus

Sigmoid sulcus

Internal occipital crest

Groove for transverse sinus

Internal occipital protuberance

Fig. 7L: Middle and posterior part of the norma basalis interna

- The *foramen lacerum* is situated postero-medial to foramen ovale, between the body of sphenoid and apex of petrous temporal bone. The carotid canal opens in its posterolateral part. The carotid artery traverses the upper part of foramen lacerum. The pterygoid canal opens in its anterior margin and gives passage to the nerve of pterygoid canal.
- In the lateral part of the floor the *markings of the middle meningeal vessels* are seen. The groove runs forward and laterally from the foramen spinosum and later divides into two for anterior and posterior branches of middle meningeal artery.
- The anterior surface of the *petrous temporal bone* forms the posterior wall of the middle cranial fossa. Near the apex, a shallow depression is seen. It is known as *trigeminal impression* for the trigeminal ganglion. *Arcuate eminence* is a prominent elevation deep to which lies the superior semicircular canal. The area lateral to the eminence is formed by the thin plate of bone called as *tegmen tympani.* This forms the roof of middle ear cavity and auditory tube. The anterior surface of the petrous temporal bone presents two grooves running downwards and medially. The upper and medial groove begins at the hiatus for greater superficial petrosal nerve and runs towards the foramen lacerum. It lodges greater superficial petrosal nerve. The lower and lateral groove begins at hiatus for lesser petrosal nerve and runs towards foramen ovale. It lodges lesser petrosal nerve.
- The superior border of petrous bone is grooved for the lodgement of the superior petrosal sinus. Near the apex of the petrous temporal bone this border is crossed by trigeminal nerve. This border also gives attachment to the tentorium cerebelli.

Posterior Cranial Fossa

The posterior cranial fossa is the deepest of the three fossae and lodges the hind brain (cerebellum, pons and medulla).

Bones Forming the Posterior Cranial Fossa

- Posterior part of the body of sphenoid.
- Occipital bone.
- Posterior surface of petrous temporal bone.
- Mastoid part of temporal bone.
- Posteroinferior angle of parietal bone.

Sutures and Fissures of the Posterior Cranial Fossa

- The lower end of lambdoid suture. between parietal and occiptal bone.
- The parieto-mastoid suture.
- The occipito-mastoid suture.
- Petro-occipital suture.

Boundaries

The middle and posterior cranial fossa are separated from each other by the dorsum sellae, posterior clinoid process and superior border of the petrous temporal bone. On the lateral side this fossa is bounded by the mastoid part of the temporal bone and the postero-inferior angle of the parietal bone. Posteriorly, it is bounded by the squamous part of the occipital bone.

The Floor of the Posterior Cranial Fossa

The floor can be divided in median and lateral parts (Fig. 7.36).

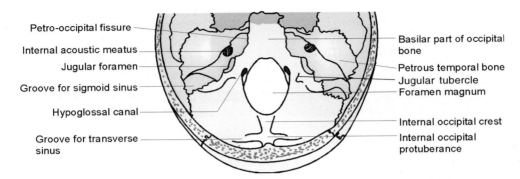

Fig. 7.36: The floor of the posterior cranial fossa. The adjacent part of middle cranial fossa is also shown

The Median Part of the Floor

The median part of the floor presents the most striking structure, i.e., the foramen magnum. The part anterior to the foramen magnum is called as clivus. The parts posterior to the foramen magnum are internal occipital crest and internal occipital protuberance.

- The *clivus* is sloping surface of the bone formed by the fusion of the basal part of the occipital bone and the body of the sphenoid. The lateral border of the basilar part of the occipital bone is separated by the petrous temporal bone by petro-occipital fissure, which lodges the inferior petrosal sinus (Fig. 7.36). The basilar part of the clivus gives attachment to the membrana tectoria, upper band of cruciate ligament and apical ligament of dens.
- The *foramen magnum* is a large oval shaped central opening in the floor of the posterior fossa. Structures passing through this foramen are shown in Fig. 7.29. On each side of the foramen magnum, the inner opening of the *hypoglossal canal* lies just above its lateral margin. It transmits the hypoglossal nerves and vessels. The *jugular tubercle* is situated between the jugular foramen and hypoglossal canal. It is related to the 9th,

10th and 11th cranial nerves. Sometimes the posterior condylar canal is also present behind the jugular foramen and lateral to the jugular tubercle. It transmits the emissary vein.

FURTHER DETAILS

Endocranial Volume and Area of Foramen Magnum

It has been reported that there exists an adequate correlation between endocranial volume and area of foramen magnum, in homonoids and mammals, which enable an accurate prediction of one quantity form the other. However, study by Routal et al. (1984) in human skulls, resulted in the finding that there is only a partial positive correlation (r=0.28) between two parameters. Hence, in human, one parameter cannot be accurately predicted from the other.

- The *internal occipital crest* is a ridge present in midline, which extends between foramen magnum and internal occipital protuberance. It gives attachment to the falx cerebelli.
- The *internal occipital protuberance* is situated opposite the external occipital protuberance. On each side it is related the

transverse sinus. It is also related to the confluence of dural venous sinuses.

The Lateral Part of the Floor (Table 7.2)

• The posterior surface of the petrous temporal bone, in its middle, shows the opening of the *internal acoustic meatus*. It transmits the facial and vestibulocochlear nerves and labyrinthine vessels. Postero-lateral to the internal meatus there lies an

Name of foramen	Structure(s) passing
	**Table 7.2: Structures passing through various foramina of the floor of cranial fossae**
Anterior Cranial Fossa	
1. Foramen caecum	Vein from nasal mucosa to superior sagittal sinus.
2. Cribriform plate	Olfactory nerves from nasal mucosa to olfactory bulb.
3. Anterior ethmoidal canal	Anterior ethmoidal nerves and vessels.
4. Posterior ethmoidal canal	Posterior ethmoidal nerves and vessels.
Middle Cranial Fossa	
5. Optic canal	Optic nerve, meninges and ophthalmic artery (Fig. 7.37).
6. Superior orbital fissure	*Lateral part*—Lacrimal nerve, frontal nerve, trochlear nerve superior ophthalmic vein, meningeal branch of lacrimal artery (Fig. 7.35).
	Middle part—Superior and inferior divisions of oculomotor nerve, nasociliary nerve and abducent nerve.
	Medial part—Inferior ophthalmic vein.
7. Foramen rotundum	Maxillary nerve.
8. Foramen ovale	Mandibular nerve, accessory meningeal artery, emissary vein and lesser petrosal nerve.
9. Foramen spinosum	Middle meningeal artery, emissary vein and meningeal branch of mandibular nerve.
10. Emissary sphenoidal f.	Emissary vein.
11. Canalis innominatus	If present it transmits lesser petrosal nerve.
12. Foramen lacerum	Ascending pharyngeal artery and emissary veins.
13. Hitus for G. petrosal nerve	Greater petrosal nerve.
14. Hitus for L. petrosal nerve	Lesser petrosal nerve.
Posterior Cranial Fossa	
15. Internal acoustic meatus	Facial and vestibulo-cochlear nerves and labyrinthine vessels.
16. Jugular foramen	*Anterior part*—Inferior petrosal sinus (Fig. 7.30).
	Middle part—Glossopharyngeal, vagus and accessory nerve.
	Posterior part—Sigmoid sinus and meningeal branch of occipital artery.
17. Foramen magnum	*Anterior part*—Apical ligament of dens, superior band of cruciate ligament and membrana tectoria.
	Posterior part—Medulla, meninges, spinal root of accessory nerve, vertebral arteries, anterior and posterior spinal arteries, tonsils of cerebellum (Fig. 7.29).
18. Hypoglossal canal	Hypoglossal nerve, emissary vein and meningeal branch of ascending pharyngeal artery.
19. Post. condylar canal	Emissary vein.

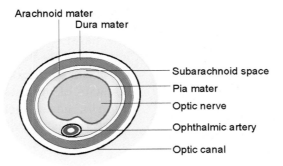

Fig. 7.37: Structure passing through optic canal

Table 7.3: Structures passing through the base of the skull (Norma basalis externa)

	Foramen/Fissure	Structures passing
1.	Incisive fossa	Greater palatine vessels and naso-palatine nerves.
2.	Greater palatine foramen	Greater palatine vessels and nerves.
3.	Lesser palatine foramen	Lesser palatine nerves and vessels.
4.	Inferior orbital fissure	Maxillary nerve, zygomatic nerve, infraorbital vessels and emissary veins (Fig. 7.38).
5.	Vomero-vaginal canal	Branches of pharyngeal nerves and vessels.
6.	Palatino-vaginal canal	Branches of pharyngeal vessels and nerves.
7.	Foramen ovale	Refer Table 7.2.
8.	Foramen spinosum	Refer Table 7.2.
9.	Foramen lacerum	Refer Table 7.2.
10.	Carotid canal	Internal carotid artery with its sympathetic and venous plexus.
11.	Petrotympanic fissure	Chorda tympani nerve, anterior lig. of malleus and ant. tympanic artery.
12.	Ant. condylar canal	Refer Table 7.2.
13.	Post. condylar canal	Refer Table 7.2.
14.	Jugular foramen	Refer Table 7.2.
15.	Foramen magnum	Refer Table 7.2.
16.	Stylomastoid foramen	Facial nerve and stylomastoid artery.

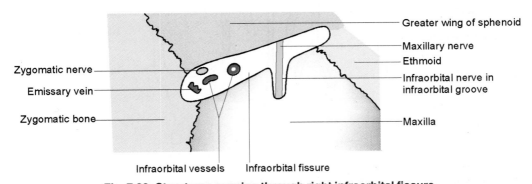

Fig. 7.38: Structures passing through right infraorbital fissure

oblique slit which leads upwards into a canal called as the aqueduct of the vestibule. It lodges succus and ductus endolymphaticus.

- The right and left transverse sulci run laterally from each side of the internal occipital protuberance. The right sulcus is more prominent. The transverse sulcus lodges transverse sinus.

- Each transverse sulcus curves downwards at the mastoid angle of parietal bone as *sigmoid sulcus*. The sigmoid sulcus runs downwards and medially with an S shaped curve. It grooves the petrous and mastoid part of the temporal bone to reach the posterior end of jugular foramen.

- The jugular foramen is situated between the posterior end of petro-occipital fissure and the terminal end of sigmoid sulcus. Above it is bounded by the petrous temporal bone and below by the jugular process of the occipital bone. It is divided into anterior, middle and posterior part (Fig. 7.30).

NASAL CAVITY

The nasal cavity is divided into right and left halves by vertical median septum (i.e., the nasal septum). Each half of the cavity consists of an anterior opening, i.e., the anterior nasal aperture, a posterior nasal aperture, lateral wall, medial wall, roof and floor (Fig. 7.39).

Anterior and Posterior Nasal Apertures

The anterior nasal apertures open on the norma frontalis (Fig.7.40), while both posterior nasal aperture opens on the base of the skull just above the posterior margin of the bony palate (Fig. 7.41).

The Medial Wall

The medial wall, anterosuperiorly, is formed by the *perpendicular plate of ethmoid*. While posteroinferiorly it is formed by the *vomer bone*. In the living condition the anterior gap in the bony septum is filled by *septal cartilage* (Fig. 7.42).

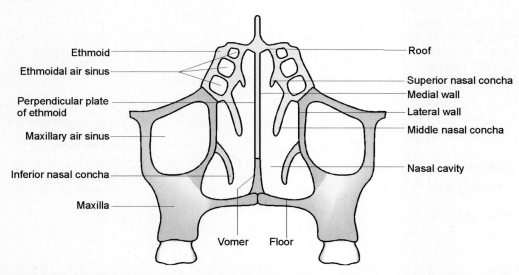

Fig. 7.39: Schematic diagram showing roof, floor, medial and lateral walls of nasal cavity (coronal section)

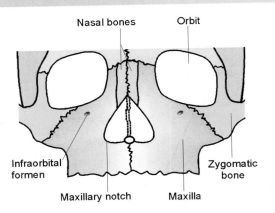

Fig. 7.40: Figure showing margins of anterior nasal aperture

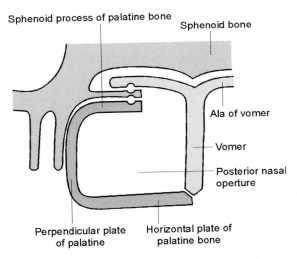

Fig. 7.41: Schematic diagram showing the bones forming posterior nasal aperture

The Lateral Wall

The lateral wall is formed by three irregular bony projections, i.e., *superior, middle and inferior conchae*. These conchae run antero-posteriorly and lie one above the other (Fig. 7.43). The spaces deep to the chonchae are called *meatuses*, i.e., superior, middle and inferior meatuses. The area above the superior concha is called as sphenoethmoidal recess. Following bones form the lateral wall of the nose:

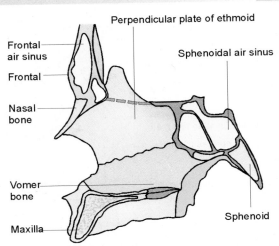

Fig. 7.42: The medial wall of the nasal cavity

- *Ethmoid*—The superior and middle conchae are the part of ethmoid bone.
- Inferior concha is a separate bone.
- Perpendicular plate of the palatine bone.
- *Maxilla*—All the above three bones are attached to the nasal surface of maxilla. A part of nasal surface of maxilla still remains free on the anterior and inferior part of the lateral wall of the nose.

Roof

From anterior to posterior, the roof is formed by nasal bone, frontal bone, cribriform plate of ethmoid, anterior surface of body of sphenoid and ala of vomer. The nasal cavity communicates with the anterior cranial fossa through numerous apertures in the cribriform plate of ethmoid bone (Fig. 7.43).

Floor

It is formed by the palatine process of the maxilla and horizontal plate of palatine bone (Fig. 7.43). In the anterior part of the floor there is the upper opening of the incisive canal.

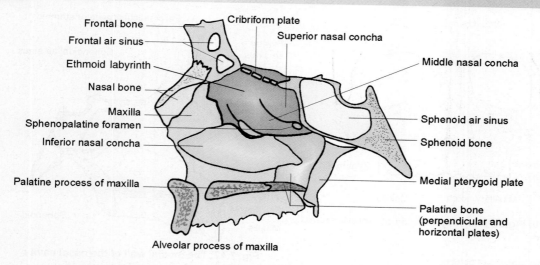

Fig. 7.43A: The lateral wall of nasal cavity as seen before removal of nasal conchae

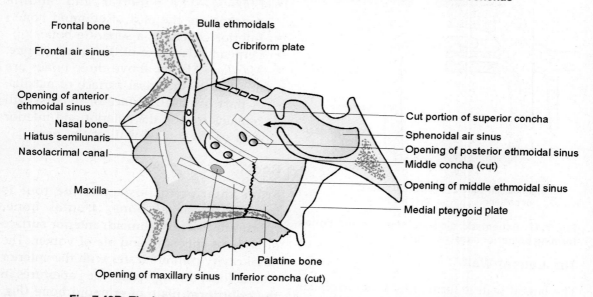

Fig. 7.43B: The lateral wall of nasal cavity as seen after removal of nasal conchae

Further Details of Lateral Wall

Sphenoethmoidal Recess

It is situated above the superior concha and receives the opening of sphenoid air sinus.

Superior Meatus

It is situated between superior and middle conchae. It receives the opening of the posterior ethmoidal sinuses.

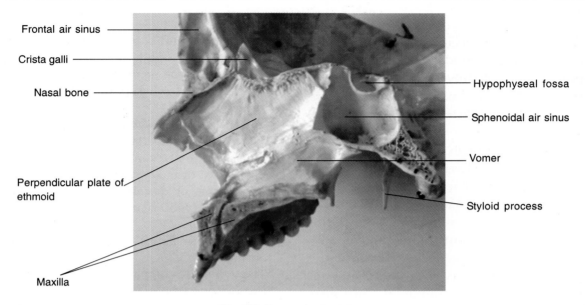

Frontal air sinus

Crista galli

Nasal bone

Perpendicular plate of ethmoid

Maxilla

Hypophyseal fossa

Sphenoidal air sinus

Vomer

Styloid process

Fig. 7M: Bony nasal septum

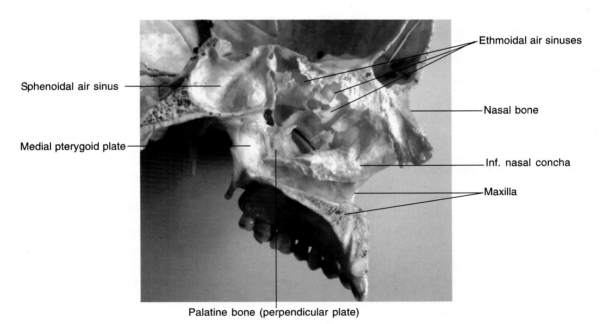

Sphenoidal air sinus

Medial pterygoid plate

Ethmoidal air sinuses

Nasal bone

Inf. nasal concha

Maxilla

Palatine bone (perpendicular plate)

Fig. 7N: Lateral bony wall of nasal cavity

Middle Meatus

It is situated between middle and inferior conchae. Deep to middle concha is a rounded prominence called the *bulla ethmoidale*. It is produced by the middle ethmoidal air sinuses. The middle ethmoidal sinuses open on the bulla.

Antero-inferior to the bulla is a curved plate of bone called as *uncinate process*. It runs downwards and backwards. The curved space between uncinate process and bulla is called as *hiatus semilunaris*. The hiatus semilunaris is continuous above and anteriorly into *infundibulum*. The infundibulum is continuous with the frontal air sinus. The anterior ethmoidal sinus also opens in the infundibulum. The maxillary air sinus opens behind the bulla at the posterior end of hiatus semilunaris.

Inferior Meatus

It is present deep to inferior concha and receives the opening of naso-lacrimal duct.

Sphenopalatine Foramen

It is present behind the superior concha and transmits sphenopalatine artery and nasal branches of pterygopalatine ganglion (Fig. 7.43).

SKULL OF THE NEWBORN

The size of the cranium (brain box) is larger as compared to the facial skeleton. The brain box (calvaria) is large because of the rapid growth of cerebrum. The bones of the vault are ossified in membrane while the bones of the base of skull are ossified in cartilage. The size of the face at birth is small due to the following facts:

Norma Frontalis

- The glabella and supercilliary arches are not well developed.
- The frontal bone is present in two halves, i.e., right and left separated by frontal suture (Fig. 7.44).
- Small size of mandible and maxilla.
- Rudimentary maxillary air sinus.
- Non-eruption of teeth.
- Small size of nasal cavity.
- The germs of developing teeth in the superior alveolar process are near the orbital floor.
- The paranasal sinuses are rudimentary or absent.
- The two halves of mandible are united by the fibrous tissue at symphysis menti. These halves join each other at end of first year.

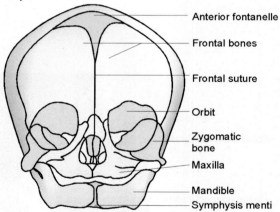

Anterior fontanelle

Frontal bones

Frontal suture

Orbit

Zygomatic bone

Maxilla

Mandible

Symphysis menti

Fig. 7.44: Skull of a newborn as seen from front

The Base of the Cranium

- The cranial base is relatively short.
- Occipital and sphenoid bones are joined with each other by the cartilaginous joint.
- The squamous, lateral and basilar parts of the occipital bone are separated from each other.

- The styloid process is not fused with the temporal bone.
- The mandibular fossa is flat and its articular tubercle underdeveloped.
- The stylomastoid foramen is exposed on the lateral surface.

The Lateral View

- The mastoid process is absent (Fig. 7.45A).
- The tympanic plate is represented by a C shaped plate.
- The tympanic membrane is attached obliquely and exposed as the bony part of external acoustic meatus is yet not developed.
- The cavities of internal ear, middle ear, mastoid antrum and three ear ossicles are of adult size at birth. However, the petrous temporal bone is much small.
- The angle of the mandible is obtuse (140 degrees).
- The coronoid process is above the level of head of mandible.

Norma Verticalis

- The bones of the vault are ossified in membrane.
- The angles of the parietal bones are still membranous. Thus there are six fontanelles at four angles of both the parietal bones.
- The unpaired median fontanelles are called *anterior* and *posterior fontanelles.*
- Two lateral pairs of fontanelles are *sphenoidal* and *mastoid fontanelle.*
- The anterior fontanelle lies at the junction of sagittal, coronal and frontal sutures.
- The posterior fontanelle lies at the junction of sagittal and lambdoid sutures.
- The sphenoidal and mastoid fontanelles are at the sphenoidal and mastoid angles of the parietal bones.

Anterior Fontanelle

The anterior fontanelle is present at the junction of frontal, coronal and sagittal sutures hence, diamond shaped (Fig. 7.45). It measures about 4 cm in anteroposterior and 2.5 cm in transverse dimensions. Deep to the anterior fontanelle lies superior sagittal sinus. It is usually closed between 18 months and 2 years of age.

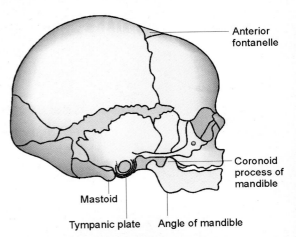

Fig. 7.45A: Newborn skull as seen from lateral aspect

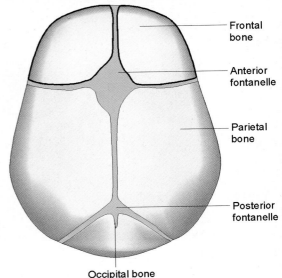

Fig. 7.45B: Newborn skull as seen from above

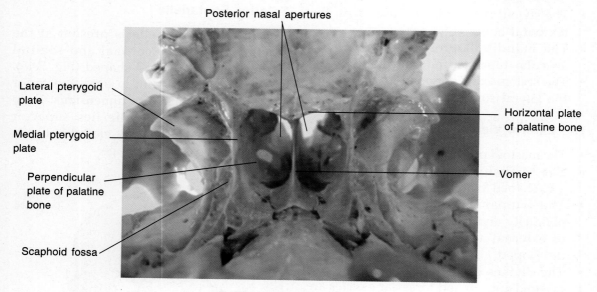

Fig. 7O: Posterior nasal aperture

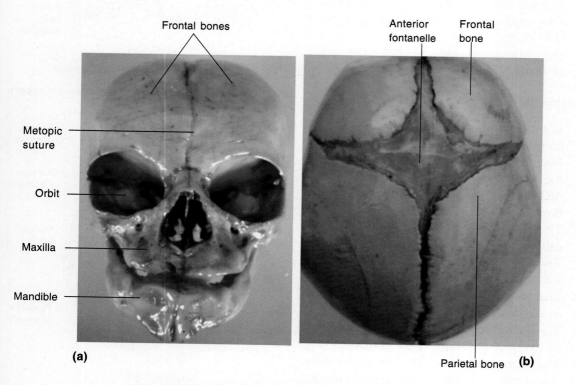

(a)

(b)

Fig. 7P: (a) Norma frontalis and (b) Norma verticalis of foetal skull

Clinical Significance

- The bulging of fontanelle indicates increased intracranial pressure.
- The depressed fontanelle indicates dehydration.
- As the superior sagittal sinus lies just deep to it blood can be withdrawn from the sinus.
- The intravenous transfusion of fluid or drugs is also possible through superior sagittal sinus.
- The CSF can also be withdrawn from the lateral ventricle of the brain. For this a needle is introduced downwards and laterally at the lateral angle of the fontanelle.
- The fact, that the anterior fontanelle closes by the age of 2 years, is utilized to determine the age of child.
- At the time of birth fontanelle allows some overlap of the bones of the cranial vault. This help in the reduction in the size of foetal head during birth.

HYOID BONE

Hyoid is a U shaped bone present in the upper part of the neck. It is not attached to any other bone but hangs at the level of 3rd cervical vertebra with the help of muscles and ligaments. The hyoid bone consists of a central *body* and *greater* and *lesser cornua* (Fig. 7.46).

Body

The body is rectangular in shape and has an anterior and a posterior surface. The anterior surface is convex and faces antero-superiorly. A median ridge divides it into right and left halves. The posterior surface is concave and smooth.

Greater Cornua

Each end of the body is continuous posterio-laterally as greater cornu. The greater cornu is flattened. It has two surfaces (upper and lower) and two borders (medial and lateral). The posterior end of the greater cornu is enlarged to form tubercle.

Lesser Cornua

The lesser cornua are small conical projections attached to the bone at the junction of body and greater cornu on each side. Each cornu projects upwards and laterally. The lesser cornu may form a synovial joint with greater cornu.

Particular Features

Attachments of muscles on the antero-superior aspect are shown in Fig. 7.47.

Attachments of ligaments and membranes are shown in Fig. 7.48.

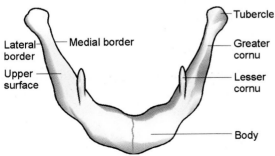

Fig. 7.46: The anterosuperior aspect of hyoid bone

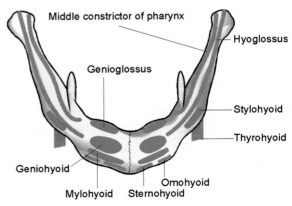

Fig. 7.47: The attachments of muscles on hyoid bone

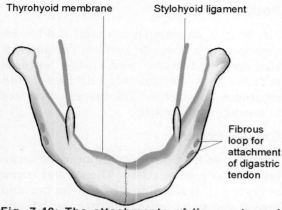

Thyrohyoid membrane   Stylohyoid ligament

Fibrous loop for attachment of digastric tendon

Fig. 7.48: The attachments of ligaments and membrane

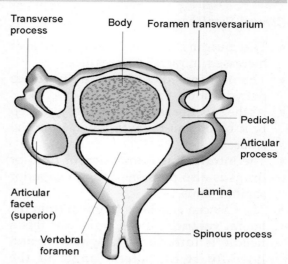

Transverse process   Body   Foramen transversarium

Pedicle

Articular process

Lamina

Spinous process

Articular facet (superior)

Vertebral foramen

Fig. 7.49: The superior aspect of a typical cervical vertebra

Ossification

The hyoid bone ossifies in cartilage by six centers. One center appears in each greater cornua at the end of intrauterine life. Soon after birth two centers appear for body. One center appears in each lesser cornua at puberty.

CERVICAL VERTEBRAE

The cervical part of the vertebral column is highly mobile and its curvature is convex anteriorly. It is made up of 7 cervical vertebrae. A cervical vertebra is characterized by the presence of a foramen in each transverse process (foramen transversarium). The 1st, 2nd and 7th vertebrae are atypical, while 3rd to 6th vertebrae are typical.

Typical Cervical Vertebrae

A typical cervical vertebra consists of body and vertebral arch (Fig. 7.49). The body and vertebral arch enclose a vertebral foramen, which lodges spinal cord and its meninges.

Body

The body of cervical vertebra is smallest among all vertebrae. The shape of the cervical vertebra is oval, its anteroposterior diameter is less than side to side.

- The superior surface of the body is concave from side to side because of the presence of upward projecting lip on either side.
- The inferior surface is convex from side to side. The anterior border of inferior surface projects downwards as a lip.
- The bodies of the adjacent vertebrae are connected by the intervertebral disc and a pair of the synovial *unconvertebral joints* on each side of the disc.
- The vertebral foramen is large and triangular is shape.

Vertebral Arch

It consists of pedicles, laminae, superior and inferior articular processes, transverse processes and spine.

Pedicles

These are rounded bar that arise from the

posterolateral part of the body. They are directed backwards and laterally hence, vertebral foramen is large and triangular.

Lamina

Laminae are thin plates of bone. They are directed backwards and medially from pedicles to meet each other in midline at the base of spinous process.

Spinous Process

It is short and bifid.

Articular Process

- The superior and inferior articular processes are present at the junction of pedicles and laminae and form a continuous articular pillar.
- The superior articular facet faces upwards and backwards while inferior facet faces downwards and forwards.
- The superior articular process articulates with the inferior articular process of the above vertebra.
- Between superior and inferior articular facets articular process is in the form of a bar and is known as *articular pillar*.
- Besides bodies the articular processes (articular pillar) also carry a considerable load of the head and neck.

Transverse Processes

- These are short and directed laterally. Each transverse process bears a foramen transversarium.
- Each process presents anterior and posterior roots (anterior and posterior to the foramen), anterior and posterior tubercles (at the lateral end of anterior

and posterior roots) and an inter-tubercular bar (costotransverse bar) which is present lateral to the foramen (Fig. 7.50).

- The anterior root, anterior tubercle, inter-tubercular bar and posterior tubercle represent the costal element (element of rib). The posterior root represent true transverse process.
- The foramen transversarium of the cervical vertebrae (except C7) transmit vertebral artery, sympathetic nerve plexus and vertebral vein.
- The upper surface of the costotransverse bar is grooved and lodges ventral ramus of corresponding cervical nerve.

The First Cervical Vertebra

The first cervical vertebra is also known as atlas. It is easily identified from the rest of the other cervical vertebrae because:

- It is ring shaped.
- It has no body.
- It is widest of all other cervical vertebrae.
- It has no spinous process.

The bone has two large masses (lateral masses) joined anteriorly by short anterior arch and joined posteriorly by a much longer

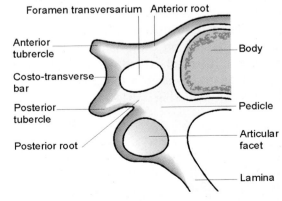

Fig. 7.50: Schematic diagram showing the parts of transverse process

posterior arch (Fig. 7.51). The superior surface of each lateral mass bear an elongated kidney shaped concave articular facet for the articulation with the occipital condyle (to form atlanto-occipital joint).

Anatomical Position

Hold the bone in such a way that the concave superior articular surface of the lateral masses face upwards. The short anterior arch should face anteriorly.

General Features

Lateral Mass

Each lateral mass has a superior articular facet and an inferior articular facet. The superior facet is concave and kidney shaped. The inferior facet is oval and flat (Fig. 7.51B). The inferior facet faces downwards and medially and articulates with the superior articular surface of the axis (2nd cervical vertebra) to form *lateral atlantoaxial joint*. The medial surface of each lateral mass bears a tubercle for the attachment of the transverse ligament of atlas.

The Anterior Arch

It shows the presence of a small anterior tubercle in the midline. An oval articular facet is present on the posterior surface in midline. This facet articulates with the dens of 2nd cervical vertebra to form the *median atlantoaxial joint* (Fig. 7.51A).

The Posterior Arch

The posterior arch is much longer than anterior and bears a posterior tubercle on its posterior surface in midline. It represents the rudimentary spinous process. There is presence of a shallow groove on its superior surface posterior to each lateral mass. The

groove lodges the vertebral artery and first cervical spinal nerve (Fig. 7.53).

The Transverse Process

The transverse process projects laterally from the lateral mass. It has foramen transversarium which transmits vertebral artery, vein and sympathetic nerve.

Particular Features

Attachments of ligaments, membranes and muscles are shown in Fig. 7.52.

Relations of blood vessels and nerves are shown in Fig. 7.53.

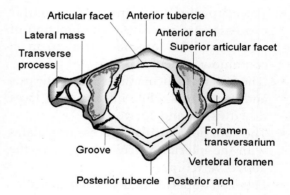

Fig. 7.51A: Superior aspect of atlas vertebra

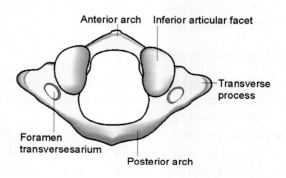

Fig. 7.51B: Inferior aspect of atlas vertebra

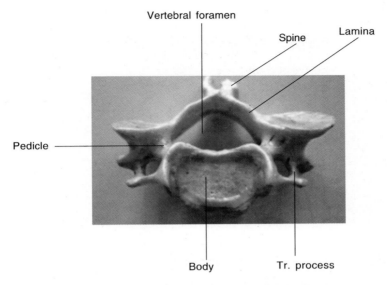

Fig. 7Q: Superior view of typical cervical vertebra

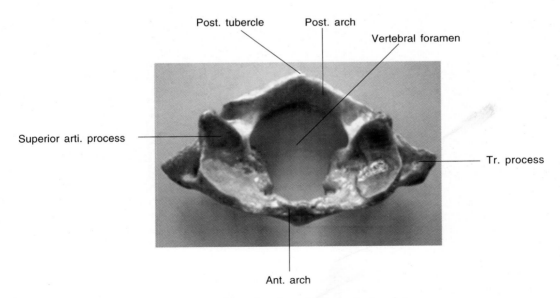

Fig. 7R: Superior view of 1st cervical vertebra

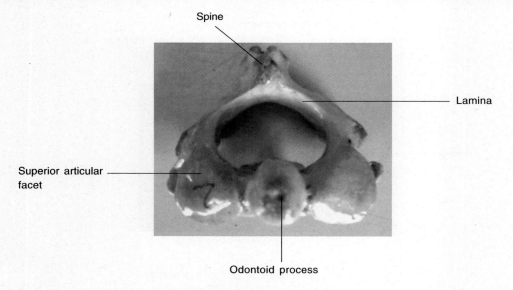

Fig. 7S: Superior view of 2nd vertebra

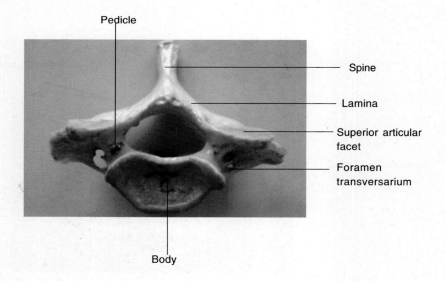

Fig. 7T: Superior view of 7th cervical vertebra

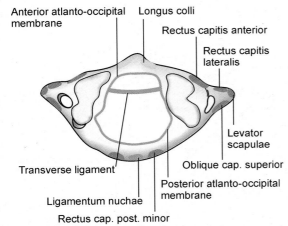

Fig. 7.52: Attachment of ligaments and membranes on superior surface of atlas

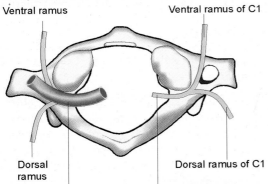

Fig. 7.53: Nerve and artery in relation to atlas. The vertebral artery is shown on left side only

The Second Cervical Vertebra

This vertebra is also known as the axis. It can be easily identified from the rest of the other vertebrae because of the presence of *dens or odontoid process*. The dens is a blunt conical tooth like process which projects superiorly from the body (Fig. 7.54). The spinous process is long, strong and bifid and projects posteriorly (Fig. 7.55).

Anatomical Position

Hold the bone in such a way that the body of the vertebra lie anteriorly and the odontoid process faces upwards. The bifid spinous process should face posteriorly.

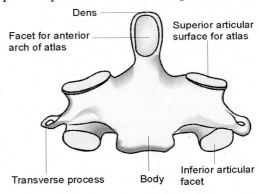

Fig. 7.54: The anterior aspect of axis vertebra

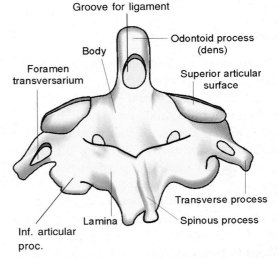

Fig. 7.55: The posterior aspect of axis vertebra

General Features

- The *odontoid process* is about 1.5 cm long. Its anterior surface bears a small oval facet for the articulation with the anterior arch of atlas (Fig. 7.54). The posterior surface shows a groove, which lodges the transverse ligament of atlas.
- The upper end of the body bears dens, while lower surface articulates with the third cervical vertebra through intervertebral disc.
- Superior articular facets are situated lateral to the odontoid process. These are large oval facets, which articulate with the corresponding inferior facets of atlas vertebra. Each facet is sloping and partly situated on the body and partly on the pedicle.
- The transverse processes are small and lie lateral to the superior articular facets.
- The pedicle, lamina and spine are massive and very strong. The spine is bifid.
- The inferior articular process is present at the junction of pedicle and lamina. Its articular facet faces downwards and forwards.

Seventh Cervical Vertebra

This vertebra is easily identified from the other cervical vertebrae due to the presence of very long, horizontal spinous process, which is not bifid (ends in a single tubercle) (Fig. 7.56). As the tip of the spinous process (tubercle) can be easily felt under the skin it is also called vertebra prominence. The transverse processes are large and have prominent posterior tubercle. The foramen transversarium is small because it does not provide passage to the vertebral artery. It transmits the accessory vertebral vein only.

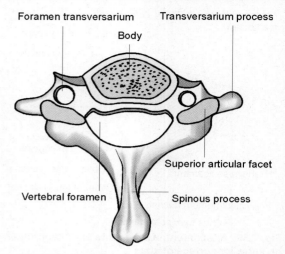

Fig. 7.56: Superior view of 7th cervical vertebra

FURTHER DETAILS

Load Transmission Through Cervical Column

According to Pal and Routal (1986), the compressive force in cervical column (from C2 to C7), is transmitted through three parallel columns—one anterior, formed by bodies and intervertebral discs, and two posterior, formed by successive articulations of the articular processes on either side. Due to posterior curvature (posterior concavity) in the cervical region, the posterior column here sustains more of the compressive force.

At C2 level the compressive force acting on two superior articular surfaces is transmitted to the inferior surface of the body and to the two inferior articular facets (Fig. 7.57). From the inferior surface of axis vertebra the compressive force is carried through three columns, anteriorly by bodies and intervertebral discs and posteriorly by articular processes (Fig. 7.58). The articular processes in cervical region are very strong bar-like structures and their articulations form strong columns posterolateral to the vertebral bodies (Fig. 7.59).

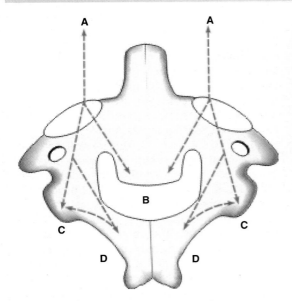

Fig. 7.57: Line diagram of the axis vertebra showing the distribution of the compressive force (A) from the superior articular surface to the body (B) and the inferior articular facets (C). Load also passes to inferior articular facet via lamina (D) (Refer Figs. 7.58 and 7.60)

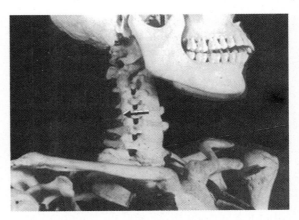

Fig. 7.59: Arrow indicating the right posterior column formed by successive articulations of articular processes

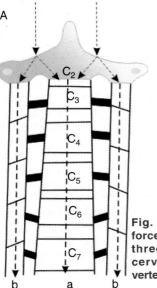

Fig. 7.58: Compressive force is carried through three columns in the cervical region of the vertebral column

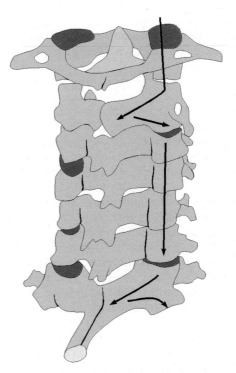

Fig. 7.60: Diagram indicating route of the axial load transmitted through the neural arches (arrows). The load becomes diffused into the laminae of C2 and C7 while it remains mostly confined to the articular pillars between C3 and C6 levels

On the basis of articular surface area it was calculated that about 54% of load passes through anterior column formed by bodies and intervertebral discs and 46% of the compressive force passes through two posterior columns (23% each).

The magnitude of load passing through three cervical columns was tested experimentally on Instron load testing machine by Pal and Sherk (1988). The experiment confirmed the presence of three weight bearing columns and the role of neural arch in transmission of vertebral compressive forces. The observation that the laminae of C2 and C7 vertebrae are thick and massive, while the laminae of C3 to C6 are very thin, prompted Pal and Routal (1996) to study the role of cervical laminae in the load transmission. Study indicated that the laminae of C2 and C7 are heavily loaded, whilst the intervening ones were not. The diffusion of load was found to be low on laminae C3 to C6. This is because, at these levels, the articular processes are in the form of a bar-like structures and form rod-like columns. Because of this reason load passing from superior to inferior articular facets are not dispersed much onto the laminae and remain confined to rod-like column. However, at C2 and C7 levels articular processes are not in the form of a bar-like structure hence, load diffuses into the lamina at C2 and C7 levels while it is being transmitted from superior to inferior articular facet (Fig. 7.60).

The observation that the lamina of C2 vertebra is involved in transmission of load from superior articular facet to inferior facet was also confirmed by trabecular bone study (Pal et al., 1988). In the lamina of axis, it was observed that the superior border of lamina is made up of thick compact bone whose thickness reduces as it turns towards the spinous process. From the border, thick bony plates run obliquely downwards and backwards towards the middle of the lamina. From the middle of the lamina, another set of plates run downwards towards the inferior facet. The superior set of plates brings the compressive forces from the superior articular surfaces to the lamina through pedicle, while lower set of plates carries this compressive force from the lamina to inferior articular facet (Fig. 7.61). Thus the lamina in the axis is involved in the transfer of compressive forces by changing their direction.

As the compressive forces are diffused on the laminae of C2 and C7, the laminectomy at these levels will result in severe cervical instability. However, due to the confinement of forces on the articular pillars between C3 and C6, laminectomy is relatively safe at these levels. On the other hand, proportion of load bearing at facet joints is remarkably uniform and the two rod-like columns are highly loaded. Therefore to minimize postoperative deformities interference with facets and articular processes is to be avoided as far as possible.

Orientation of Articular Facets in the Cervical Column

The facet joints are important structures in determining the biomechanical properties of the spinal column and are of clinical relevance. The pattern of orientation of facets guides and limits the excursion of the motion segments. Study by Pal et al. (2001) showed that all vertebrae at C3 level and 73% at C4 level displayed posteromedially facing superior articular facets. This kind of orientation of C2/C3 facet joint do not allow C2 vertebra to rotate on C3 and thus keep C2 vertebra fixed during rotational movements at atlanto-axial joint (Fig. 4.18). Similarly at T1 level (C7/T1 joint) all columns showed posterolaterally facing superior articular facets (Fig. 7.62).

The level of change in orientation, from posteromedial to posterolateral facing superior facets, was not constant and occurred anywhere between C4 (C3/C4 joint) and T1 (C7/T1 joint). The C6 (C5/C6 joint) vertebra was the most frequent site to show the transition (from posteromedial to posterolateral). The C5/C6 joint showed the wide range of a movement and was the most common site to show the bilateral facet dislocation.

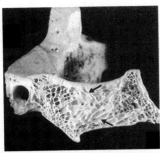

Fig. 7.61: Trabeculae in the lamina of the axis exposed after removal of the compact bone from the lateral surface. A set of bony plates is seen to run downwards and backwards from the thick compact bone at the superior border (upper arrow). Another set of parallel plates runs obliquely from the upper set towards the inferior articular facet (lower arrow)

Further Readings

- Routal R.V., Pal G.P. and Bhagwat S.S. (1984). *Journal Anatomy Soc. India,* Vol. 33(3), 145-149.
- Pal G.P., Bhagwat S.S. and Routal R.V. (1986a). *Anthrop. Anz.,* Vol. 44(1), 67-76.
- Pal G.P. and Routal R.V. (1986b). *Anthrop. Anz.,* Vol. 44 (2), 169-173.
- Pal G.P., Bhagwat S.S. and Routal R.V. (1986c). *Jou. Anat. Soc. India* 35, 115-120.
- Pal G.P. and Routal R.V. (1986). *Journal of Anatomy* (UK) 148, 245-261.
- Pal G.P. and Routal R.V. (1987). *Journal of Anatomy* (U.K.) 152, 13-105.
- Pal, G.P. Cosio L., Routal R. (1988). *Anatomical Record* (USA) 222, 418-425.
- Pal G.P. and Sherk H. (1988). *Spine* (Am. Vol.) 13(5), 447-449.
- Pal G.P., Cosio L. and Routal R.V. (1988). *The Anatomical Record* (USA) 222, 418-425.
- Pal G.P. and Routal R.V. (1996). *Journal of Anatomy* (UK) 188, 485-489.
- Pal G.P., Routal R.V. and S.K. Saggu (2001). *Journal of Anatomy* (UK) 198, 431-441.

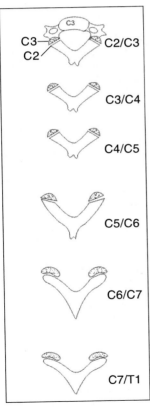

Fig. 7.62: Note that the superior articular facets of C3 are facing posteromedially while that of C6 are facing posterolaterally. The change is orientation from posteromedial to posterolateral usually occurs at C5/C6 junction

Bones of the Skull

MANDIBLE

The mandible is the bone of the lower jaw. It has a horseshoe shaped body and two broad rami projecting upwards from the posterior part of the body (Fig. 8.1). The junction between body and ramus is obtained by drawing a vertical line along the anterior border of the ramus.

General Features

Body

The body is U shaped and has two surfaces and two borders. It consists of right and left halves united in the median plane at the symphysis menti. The symphysis menti is a faint ridge on the upper part of the midline.

Upper Border

The upper border of the mandible is also known as alveolar border. It bears sockets for the teeth.

Lower Border

This border is also known as the base of the mandible. Posteriorly it is continuous with the lower border of the ramus of mandible (Fig. 8.2). On either side of midline there is the presence of digastric fossa for the attachment of the anterior belly of digastric.

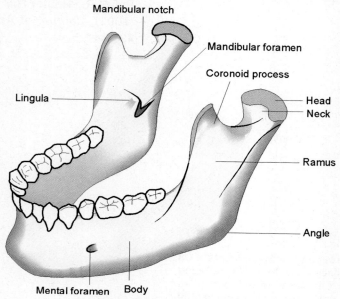

Fig. 8.1: The mandible of an adult

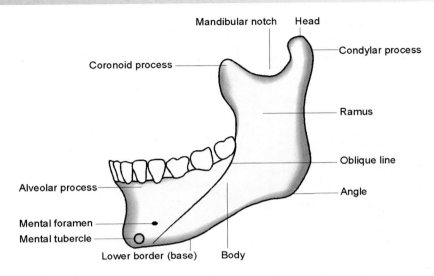

Fig. 8.2: The lateral surface of one half of the mandible

External Surface

- At the lower part of the midline (at symphysis menti) a triangular *mental protuberance* is present.
- The upper angle of the triangle lies at the lower end of symphysis menti. The *mental tubercles* are present at the lower angles of this triangle (Fig. 8.2).
- A faint ridge is present on the external surface of body extending upwards and backwards from the mental tubercle up to the anterior margin of the ramus. This is called as *oblique line*.
- The *mental foramen*, in an adult, is present below the second premolar tooth midway between upper and lower borders.

Internal Surface

- The *mylohyoid line* is an oblique line, extends diagonally downwards and forwards from just below the alveolar border (behind the 3rd molar tooth) to the lower part of symphysis menti (Fig. 8.3).
- *Sublingual fossa* is a smooth area above the anterior part of the mylohyoid line for the lodgement of sublingual salivary gland.
- The submandibular fossa is a concave area present below the posterior part of mylohyoid line. It comes in contact with the superficial part of the submandibular gland.
- The posterior part of the symphysis menti on either side of the midline presents a pair of elevations called superior and inferior *genial tubercles*. These tubercles are present above the anterior end of mylohyoid line (Fig. 8.3).

Ramus of Mandible

The ramus of the mandible projects upwards from the posterior part of the body. It has four borders (anterior, posterior, upper and lower), two surfaces (lateral and medial) and two processes (coronoid and condylar).

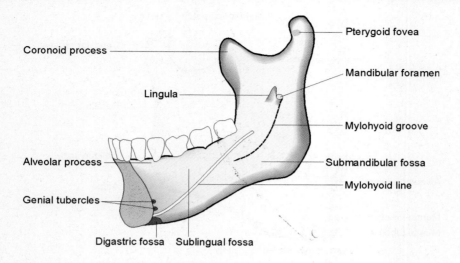

Coronoid process —

Lingula —

Alveolar process —

Genial tubercles —

Digastric fossa   Sublingual fossa

Pterygoid fovea

Mandibular foramen

Mylohyoid groove

Submandibular fossa

Mylohyoid line

Fig. 8.3: The medial surface of one half of the mandible

Borders

- The upper border forms a notch, i.e., the *mandibular notch*. This border displays a triangular *coronoid process* anteriorly and *condylar process* posteriorly (Fig. 8.2).
- The lower border is the backward continuation of the base of the body of mandible.
- The anterior border of the ramus is sharp and continuous below with the oblique line on the lateral surface of the body of mandible.
- The posterior border meets with the lower border of the ramus to form the angle of mandible. This border is in continuation above with the condylar process.

Processes

- The coronoid process is flat and triangular, which projects upwards from the antero-superior part of the ramus. It lies at the junction of upper (mandibular notch) and anterior border of ramus.
- The condylar process projects upwards

from the posterosuperior part of the ramus. The upper end of the condylar process is expanded and forms *head of the mandible*. While the lower part of the condylar process is constricted and called *neck*.

- Head of the mandible bears articular surface that articulates with the mandibular fossa of the temporal bone to form temporomandibular joint. The anterior surface of the neck shows a depression called *pterygoid fovea* for attachment of lateral pterygoid muscle.

Surfaces

- The *lateral surface* is rough and flat in its anteroinferior part for the attachment of masseter (Fig. 8.2).
- *Medial surface* presents a *mandibular foramen* close to its center (Fig. 8.3). It leads into mandibular canal which opens at the mental foramen.
- The *lingula* is a tongue shaped projection near the anterior margin of the

mandibular foramen. There is the presence of a *mylohoid groove* just behind the lingula. This groove runs forwards and downwards from the mandibular foramen to the inner surface of the body of mandible.

- The area above the angle of mandible is rough for the attachment of medial pterygoid muscle.

Particular Features

Attachments of muscles are shown in Fig. 8.4 for extenal surface and in Fig. 8.5 for internal surface.

Relations of nerves, blood vessels, glands and ligaments are shown in Fig. 8.6.

Ossification

The part of the bone between mental foramen and mandibular foramen ossify in membrane (fibrous envelop of the Meckel's cartilage of first branchial arch). The part of the body in front of the mental foramen and the part of ramus above mandibular foramen ossify in cartilage (Fig. 8.7). Each half of mandible ossify in 6th week of IUL. At birth mandible consists of two halves of the mandibular

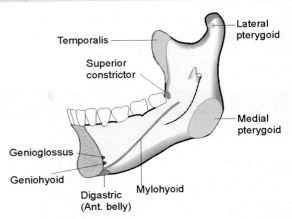

Fig. 8.5: Attachments of muscles on the internal surface of mandible

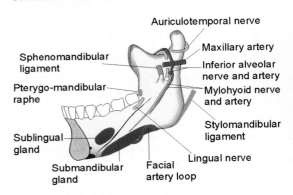

Fig. 8.6: Figure showing relations of nerves, blood vessels, glands and ligaments on the medial aspect of mandible

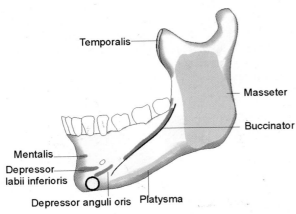

Fig. 8.4: The attachments of muscles on the external surface of mandible

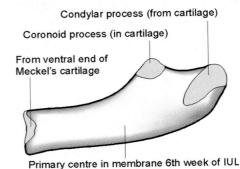

Fig. 8.7: Figure showing the ossification of left half of mandible. Yellow area shows the bone developing from membrane. The coronoid, condylar process and the area of genial tubercles develops from cartilagenous ossification (shown in blue)

body united by the fibrous joint at symphysis menti. This fibrous joint is replaced by bony union at the end of first year of postnatal age.

Age Changes in Mandible

The bony features of mandible change with age (children, adult and old age). For detail refer Table 8.1 and Fig. 8.8.

Table 8.1: Age changes in mandible			
Teeth	Mandibular canal and mental foramen	Angle of the mandible	Level of the condylar and coronoid process
Children			
Milk and permanent teeth are present in mandible.	Both mental foramen and canal lies close to lower border because of the presence of both deciduous and permanent teeth in the body of mandible. The opening of foramen is directed forwards.	It is obtuse (140 degrees).	The coronoid process is above the level of condylar process.
Adult			
All the permanent teeth are present.	Due to subalveolar deposition of bone (at the lower border) the mental foramen is midway between upper and lower borders. The foramen opens backwards. Mandibular canal runs almost parallel to the mylohyoid line.	It is between 110 to 115 degrees due to the posterior growth of ramus.	Condylar process is above the level of coronoid process.
Old Age			
Loss of permanent teeth.	The mental foramen and canal shift near the upper border due to loss of teeth and alveolar bone. The foramen opens backwards.	It is obtuse again (140).This is part of an old age adaptation to enable the contact between upper and lower jaws.	Coronoid process is slightly above the condylar process due to appearance of a backward bend in the neck.

Fig. 8.8: Age changes in mandible

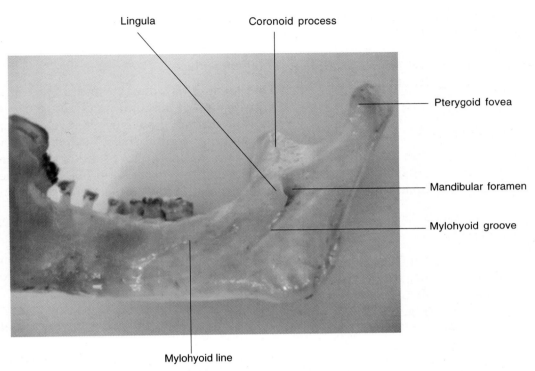

Lingula

Coronoid process

Pterygoid fovea

Mandibular foramen

Mylohyoid groove

Mylohyoid line

Fig. 8A: Internal surface of body and ramus of mandible

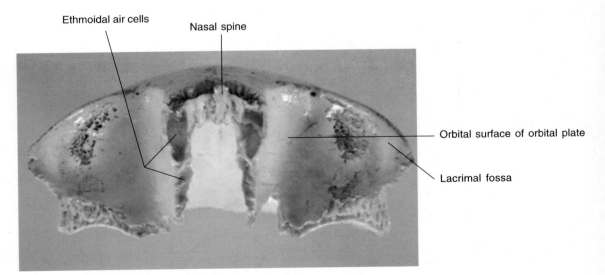

Ethmoidal air cells

Nasal spine

Orbital surface of orbital plate

Lacrimal fossa

Fig. 8B: Inferior surface of frontal bone

FRONTAL BONE

Frontal bone forms the most of the part of anterior cranial fossa. The bone consists of *squamous (main)* part and *orbital parts.* The squamous part forms forehead and orbital parts form the major part of the roof of each orbit.

Squamous (Main) Part

This part of the bone has got an external surface and internal surface, right and left temporal surface, nasal part and zygomatic processes.

External Surface

The external surface of the squamous part forms the forehead. This surface presents frontal eminence about 3 cms above the supraorbital margin (Fig. 8.9). The other features seen on this surface are glabella, superciliary arches and supraorbital margins. The supraorbital notch or foramen is seen on the supraorbital margin. Occasionally the metopic suture may be seen in the region of glabella.

Temporal Surface

This forms a small surface on the right and left sides below the temporal lines.

Internal Surface

This surface is concave and shows the impressions of cerebral sulci and gyri. It shows a median groove (sagittal sulcus) for the superior sagittal sinus. At the anterior end of groove there is presence of a median ridge called the *frontal crest.* Just below the frontal crest is the presence of foramen caecum.

Nasal Part

The nasal part is the downward projection of squamous part of bone between two superior orbital margins.
- The lower serrated margin of this part is concave downwards and known as *nasal notch.*
- The nasal notch bears a median projection, the *nasal spine* which articulates with the nasal bones in front and behind with the perpendicular plate of ethmoid.

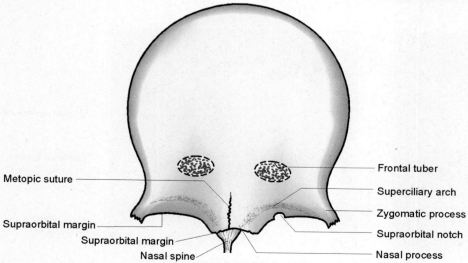

Fig. 8.9: Frontal bone as seen from external aspect

- From medial to lateral, the nasal bone, frontal process of maxilla and lacrimal bone articulate with each half of the nasal notch.

Zygomatic Process

The zygomatic process passes downwards and laterally from the lateral end of superior orbital margin.

The Orbital Part

The orbital part consists of right and left orbital plates separated from each other by a wide notch called *ethmoid notch* (Fig. 8.10).
- The notch is occupied by the ethmoid bone.
- The orbital surface faces downwards. It is smooth and forms the roof of the orbit.
- The inferior aspect of the orbital plate, just lateral to notch, shows the depressions of ethmoidal air cells. More anteriorly it shows the opening of frontal air sinus.

- There is presence of *lacrimal fossa* at its anterolateral angle.
- The *trochlear fovea* is present, at its antero-medial part.
- The upper surface of the orbital plate forms the floor of the anterior cranial fossa and shows the impressions for sulci and gyri.

Articulations

Following bones articulate with the squamous part of the frontal bone:

Posteriorly: Parietal bones (at the coronal suture), greater wings of sphenoid.

Anteriorly: Zygomatic bone, nasal bone, frontal process of maxilla, lacrimal bone and perpendicular plate of ethmoid.

Following bones articulate with the orbital part:

Posteriorly: Lesser wings of sphenoid.
Medially: Orbital plate of ethmoid.

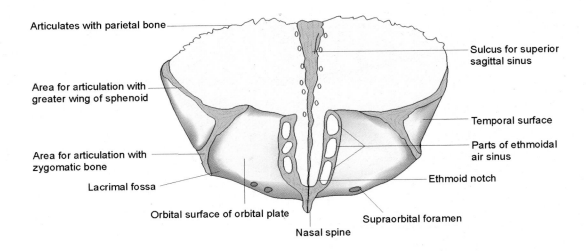

Fig. 8.10: Frontal bone as seen from inferior aspect

Ossification

It ossifies in membrane (Fig. 8.11).

Two halves of frontal bone begin to fuse at the age of first post natal year. The fusion is completed by the end of eight years. If the suture persists in adults then it is known as *metopic suture.*

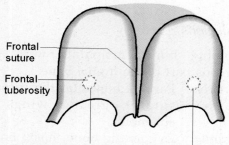

Frontal suture

Frontal tuberosity

Primary centre in membrane (8th week of IUL)

Fig. 8.11: The ossification of frontal bone. The bone as seen in newborn

PARIETAL BONE

The parietal bones are quadrilateral in shape

and form the roof and side walls of the cranial cavity.

General Features

Each bone has:

Four borders: Superior, inferior, anterior and posterior.

Two surfaces: External and internal.

Four angles: Anterosuperior, anteroinferior, posterosuperior and postero-inferior.

The *external surface* is convex. The external surface shows the parietal eminence, parietal foramen and superior and inferior temporal lines (Fig. 8.12).

On the concave *internal surface* the vascular grooves (for middle meningeal vessels) run upwards and backwards from the antero-inferior angle. A shallow groove for sigmoid sinus is seen at its postero-inferior angle (Fig. 8.13).

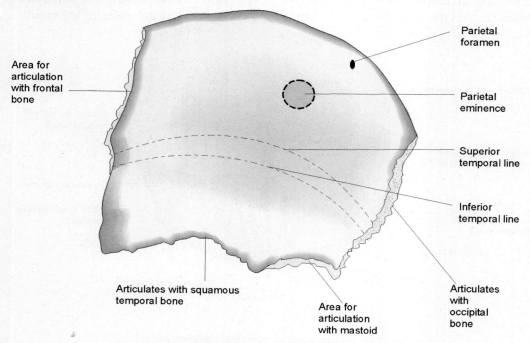

Parietal foramen

Area for articulation with frontal bone

Parietal eminence

Superior temporal line

Inferior temporal line

Articulates with squamous temporal bone

Area for articulation with mastoid

Articulates with occipital bone

Fig. 8.12: The external surface of left parietal bone

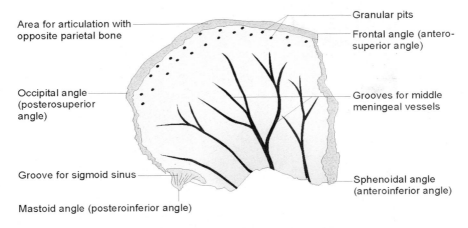

Area for articulation with opposite parietal bone

Granular pits

Frontal angle (antero-superior angle)

Occipital angle (posterosuperior angle)

Grooves for middle meningeal vessels

Groove for sigmoid sinus

Sphenoidal angle (anteroinferior angle)

Mastoid angle (posteroinferior angle)

Fig. 8.13: The internal surface of left parietal bone

Particular Features

The attachments and relations of the bone with the soft tissues are shown in Figs. 8.14 and 8.15.

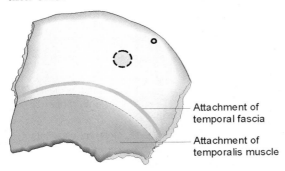

Attachment of temporal fascia

Attachment of temporalis muscle

Fig. 8.14: Attachments on left parietal bone

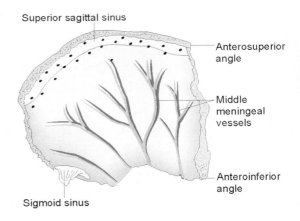

Superior sagittal sinus

Anterosuperior angle

Middle meningeal vessels

Anteroinferior angle

Sigmoid sinus

Fig. 8.15: Blood vessels and sinus in relation to the internal surface of left parietal bone

Articulations

Articulations of parietal bone are shown in Fig. 8.12.

Side Determination

Hold the bone in such a way that convex external surface faces laterally. The angle showing vascular groove at the internal surface should be kept antero-inferiorly.

Anatomical Position

The superior border should be kept towards the median plane, the antero-inferior angle downwards and forwards.

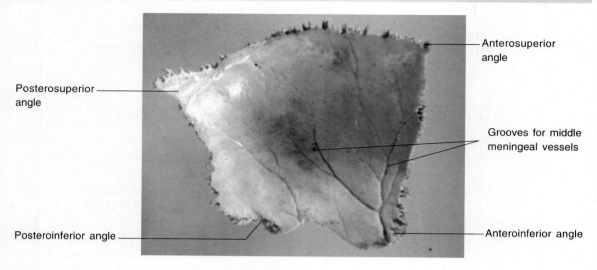

Posterosuperior angle

Anterosuperior angle

Grooves for middle meningeal vessels

Posteroinferior angle

Anteroinferior angle

Fig. 8C: Internal surface of the left parietal bone

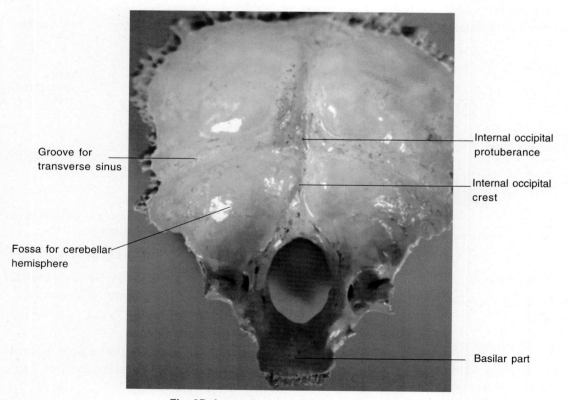

Groove for transverse sinus

Internal occipital protuberance

Internal occipital crest

Fossa for cerebellar hemisphere

Basilar part

Fig. 8D: Internal surface of the occipital bone

Ossification

It ossifies in membrane (Fig. 8.16).

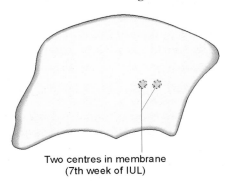

Two centres in membrane
(7th week of IUL)

Fig. 8.16: Ossification of parietal bone

OCCIPITAL BONE

This bone is present in the posterior part of the skull. The presence of the large foramen magnum helps in dividing the bone into four parts (Fig. 8.17).

- A part above and behind the foramen magnum is an expanded curved plate of bone, i.e., *squamous part.* It shows a superior angle and two lateral angles. Superior angle lies at lambda and each lateral angle at asterion (Refer Fig. 7.5).
- A part in front of foramen magnum is called *basilar part.*
- A pair of *condylar parts* is present on either side of foramen magnum (Fig. 8.17).

Anatomical Position

Hold the bone in such a way that foramen magnum should lie in the horizontal plane and basilar part should be directed forwards and upwards.

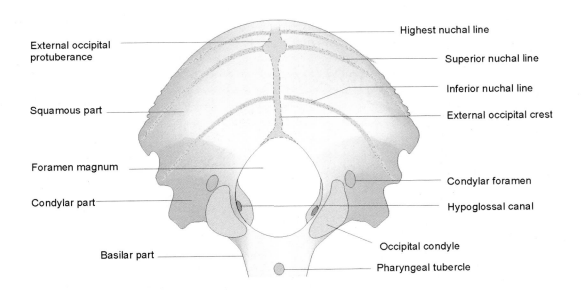

Fig. 8.17: The occipital bone as seen from inferior aspect

General Features

Squamous Part

The squamous part shows a convex external and a concave internal surface: one superior angle and two lateral angles and two borders i.e., lambdoid and mastoid borders.

- The *external surface* shows the presence of the *external occipital protuberance and external occipital crest*. The *highest nuchal line* and *superior nuchal line* runs laterally from the external occipital protuberance, on right and left sides. The inferior nuchal line runs laterally from the middle of the external occipital crest.
- The *internal surface* of the squamous part shows the presence of *internal occipital protuberance* in middle (Fig. 8.18). A wide median groove for superior sagittal sinus is present above the protuberance. Grooves for transverse sinuses are present on either side of the protuberance. An internal occipital crest runs

downwards in midline from the internal occipital protuberance.
- *Borders*—The lambdoid border articulates with the parietal bone at the lambdoid suture and mastoid border articulates with the mastoid bone at the occipito-mastoid suture (Fig. 7.19).

Basilar Part of the Occipital Bone

It extends forwards and upwards from the anterior margin of foramen magnum. This part has three surfaces (anterior, superior and inferior), and two lateral borders.

- The anterior surface extends upto the body of the sphenoid bone and forms a primary cartilaginous joint (basi-sphenoid joint), which is replaced by the bone at about 25 years of age.
- The superior surface slopes downwards and backwards and forms a part of *clivus*.
- The inferior surface bears a pharyngeal tubercle.
- The lateral border of basilar part articulates with the posterior border of petrous part of temporal bone.

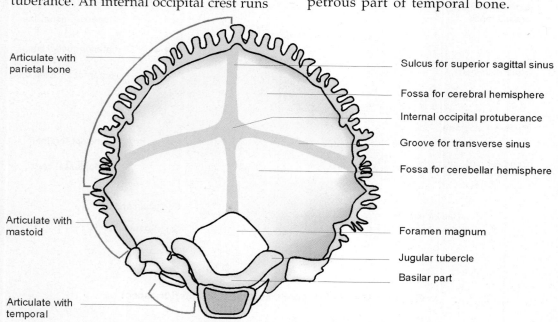

Fig. 8.18: The internal surface of the occipital bone

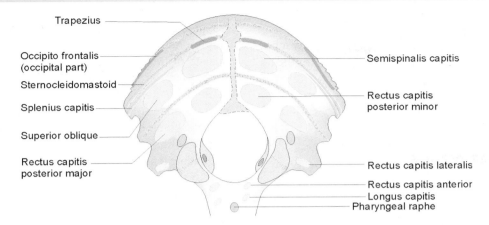

Fig. 8.19: Attachment of muscles on the inferior surface of occipital bone

Labels (clockwise): Trapezius, Occipito frontalis (occipital part), Sternocleidomastoid, Splenius capitis, Superior oblique, Rectus capitis posterior major, Semispinalis capitis, Rectus capitis posterior minor, Rectus capitis lateralis, Rectus capitis anterior, Longus capitis, Pharyngeal raphe

The Condylar Part of the Occipital Bone

It presents superior and inferior surfaces.

- The inferior surface of the condylar part presents occipital condyle. The hypoglossal or anterior condylar canal opens just above the anterolateral side of the occipital condyle. Just behind the condyle is the *condylar fossa,* which may show the opening of posterior condylar canal.
- The *jugular process* is a quadrilateral plate present lateral to the posterior half of occipital condyle. The upper surface of jugular process is deeply grooved for sigmoid sinus.
- The superior surface of condylar part shows *jugular tubercle.*

The Foramen Magnum

For structures passing through foramen magnum Fig. 7.29.

Particular Features

The soft tissue relations are shown in Figs. 8.19 and 8.20.

Articulations

Following bones articulate with the occipital bone:

Parietal (at lambdoid suture).
Mastoid (at occipitomastoid suture).
Sphenoid (at basisphenoid suture, which gets ossified about the age of 25 years).

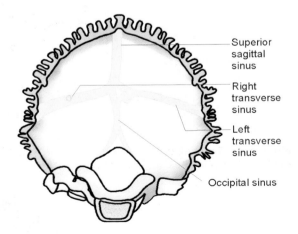

Labels: Superior sagittal sinus, Right transverse sinus, Left transverse sinus, Occipital sinus

Fig. 8.20: Dural venous sinuses in relation to squamous part of occipital bone

Ossification

The squamous part, above the highest nuchal line, ossifies in membrane. Rest of the bone ossifies in cartilage (Fig. 8.21A). The part above highest nuchal line may not unite with the rest of the bone and is then called as *interparietal bone*.

FURTHER DETAILS

Ossification of Occipital Bone

The interparietal part of the squamous occipital bone above the highest nuchal line develops in membrane. For the development of membranous part of the occipital bone, most of the authors have described two pairs of centers and an occasional third pair

(pre-interparietal) at the upper angle of the bone. Thus membranous part of the occipital bone consists of two elements, pre-interparietal and interparietal. In past, many authors believed that the preinterparietal bone is present as a separate bone at lambda. However, lambda is also the common site for the occurrence of sutural bone. Hence, it becomes difficult to differentiate a pre-interparietal bone form sutural bone at lambda.

The study by Pal *et al.* (1984) has differentiated the sutural bones at lambda from the bone developed from pre-interparietal centers. A separate pre-interparietal bone is identified by its shape and position. It is present behind the lambda (Fig. 8.21B) within the territory of the membranous occipital bone (Pal, 1987).

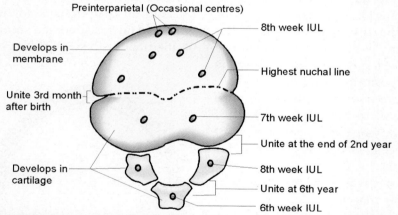

Fig. 8.21A: The ossification of occipital bone. It develops by nine centres (four in membrane and five in cartilages). Sometimes an occasional pair of centres (preinterparietal) may also appear

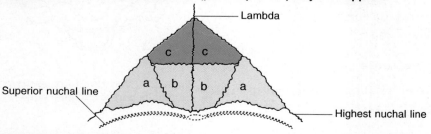

Fig. 8.21B: Diagram showing maximum variations in the interparietal region which may result due to non-fusion of three pairs of centres with each other. (a) Lateral plates; (b) Lower half of central pieces; (c) Upper half of central pieces. Upper half of central pieces develop from preinterparietal centres

ZYGOMATIC BONE

It is situated on the upper lateral part of the face and forms the prominence of the cheek. Each zygomatic bone has a *body* and two processes (a *frontal* and a *temporal* process).

General Features

The *frontal process* is directed upwards to articulate with the zygomatic process of the frontal bone. The *temporal process* extends backwards to articulate with zygomatic process of the temporal bone and forms zygomatic arch. Anteromedially the body articulates with the maxilla (Fig 8.22).

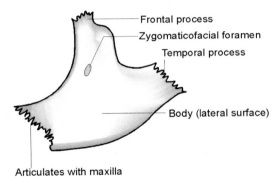

Frontal process
Zygomaticofacial foramen
Temporal process
Body (lateral surface)
Articulates with maxilla

Fig. 8.22: The external (lateral) surface of left zygomatic bone

Body

The body has three surfaces and five borders. The surfaces are *lateral, temporal* and *orbital,* while bordes are *anteroinferior, anterosuperior (orbital), posteromedial, posterosuperior and postero-inferior.*

- The *lateral surface* is convex and presents zygomaticofacial foramen. This surface forms the prominence of the cheek.
- The *orbital surface* forms the part of lateral wall and floor of orbit. It has the zygomatico-orbital foramen.

- The *temporal surface* is directed posteromedially. It forms the anterior wall of temporal fossa. The zygomatico temporal foramen is present on this surface.

Particular Features

The attachments of muscles on the zygomatic bone are shown in Fig. 8.23.

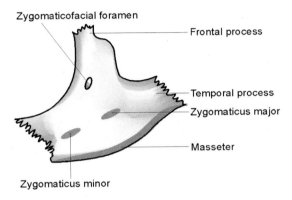

Zygomaticofacial foramen
Frontal process
Temporal process
Zygomaticus major
Masseter
Zygomaticus minor

Fig. 8.23: Attachment of muscles on zygomatic bone

Articulations

Following bones articulate with the zygomatic bone:

Frontal, maxilla, greater wing of sphenoid and zygomatic process of temporal.

Side Determination and Anatomical Position

Hold the bone in such a way that:
- The frontal process should look upwards.
- The smooth concave orbital margin should face upwards and medially.
- The smooth lateral surface should face laterally.
- The direction of lateral surface will determine the side of the bone.

Ossification

The bone ossifies in membrane (Fig. 8.24).

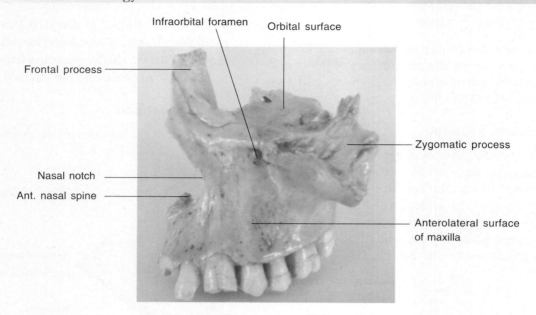

Infraorbital foramen

Orbital surface

Frontal process

Zygomatic process

Nasal notch

Ant. nasal spine

Anterolateral surface
of maxilla

Fig. 8E: Anterolateral aspect of left maxilla

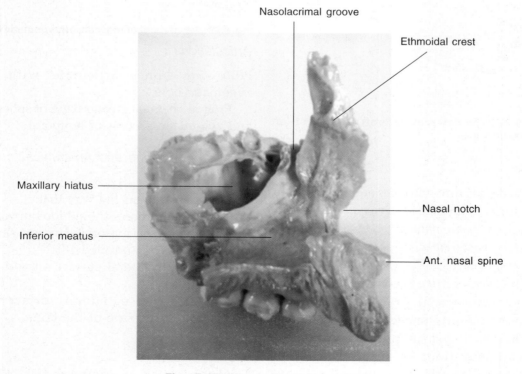

Nasolacrimal groove

Ethmoidal crest

Maxillary hiatus

Nasal notch

Inferior meatus

Ant. nasal spine

Fig. 8F: Medial aspect of left maxilla

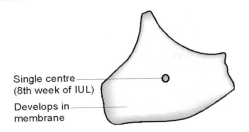

Single centre (8th week of IUL)

Develops in membrane

Fig. 8.24: Ossification of zygomatic bone, sometimes a fissure divides the bone in upper and lower parts (os japonicum)

MAXILLA

The right and left maxillae take part in the formation of the whole of the upper jaw and part of the hard palate.

General Features

Each maxilla consists of body and four processes, i.e., an alveolar process, a zygomatic process, a frontal process and a palatine process.

Body

The body is pyramidal in shape and encloses a large maxillary air sinus. Inferiorly, the body bears an alveolar process for the attachment of teeth. Body possesses four surfaces: *anterolateral, posterior, orbital and nasal.*

Anterolateral Surface

It is directed forwards and laterally. Above, the anterior surface is limited by the infraorbital margin. Medially, this surface presents a nasal notch (Fig. 8.25). Below the infraorbital margin the infraorbital foramen is present. This surface also presents canine eminence, incisive fossa and canine fossa.

Posterior Surface

It faces backwards and laterally. This surface forms the anterior wall of the infratemporal fossa hence, also known as infratemporal surface. Inferiorly, this surface shows the

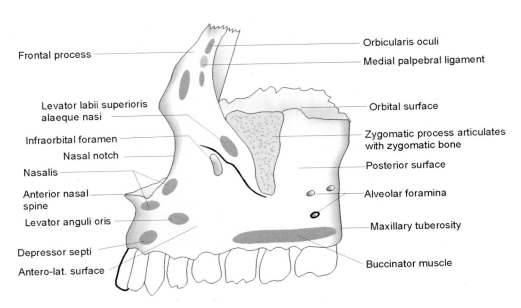

Frontal process

Levator labii superioris alaeque nasi

Infraorbital foramen

Nasal notch

Nasalis

Anterior nasal spine

Levator anguli oris

Depressor septi

Antero-lat. surface

Orbicularis oculi

Medial palpebral ligament

Orbital surface

Zygomatic process articulates with zygomatic bone

Posterior surface

Alveolar foramina

Maxillary tuberosity

Buccinator muscle

Fig. 8.25: The lateral aspect of left maxilla

maxillary tuberosity, which articulates with the pyramidal process of the palatine bone. Posterior superior alveolar foramina are seen on the surface.

Orbital Surface

It forms the major part of the floor of the orbit. Posteriorly, it forms the anteromedial border of infraorbital fissure. There is the presence of an infraorbital groove near the center of the orbital surface. This groove leads to infraorbital canal anteriorly, which opens on the anterior surface as infraorbital foramen (Fig. 8.25).

Nasal (Medial) Surface

This surface takes part in the formation of the lateral wall of the nasal cavity.
* The maxiallry air sinus opens on this surface as a large maxillary hiatus (Fig. 8.26).
* Posterior to the hiatus there is a groove, which is converted into greater palatine

canal by the perpendicular plate of palatine bone.
* Anteroinferior to the hiatus is the area of inferior meatus.
* Superior to the inferior meatus is the *nasolacrimal groove.*
* There is the presence of a ridge anterior to the nasolacrimal groove. It is called *conchal crest*, which articulates with the inferior nasal concha.

Processes

Zygomatic Process

This strong process extends laterally from the body to articulate with the body of the zygomatic bone (Fig. 8.25).

Frontal Process

It extends upwards and medially where its tip articulates with the nasal part of the frontal bone. Anteriorly this process articulates with the nasal bone and posteriorly with the lacrimal bone. The

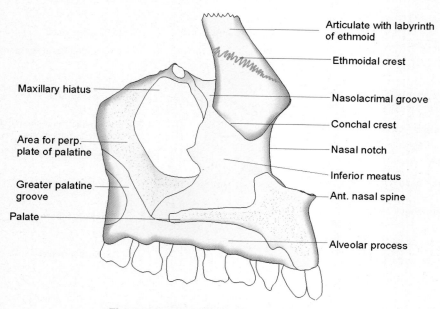

Fig. 8.26: The medial aspect of left maxilla

lateral surface of this process bears a ridge called as lacrimal crest. The medial surface is marked by an ethmoidal crest (Fig. 8.26).

Alveolar Process

It extends downwards and carries the sockets for teeth of upper jaw.

Palatine Process

It is a horizontal plate, which projects medially from the nasal surface of the body of maxilla. Medially it articulates with the palatine process of the opposite maxilla to form anterior ¾ of hard palate. It has superior and inferior surfaces and two free borders, i.e., medial and posterior. Posteriorly, it articulates with the anterior border of horizontal plate of palatine bone.

Anatomical Position and Side Determination

Hold the bone in such a way that:
• The medial border of its palatine process should be in median plane.
• The frontal process should point upwards.
• Zygomatic process laterally.

Ossification

It ossifies in membrane from a single centre which appears in 6th week of IUL.

ETHMOID

It is a single, irregular midline bone situated between two orbits, in the ethmoidal notch of the frontal bone.

The parts of the ethmoid can be appreciated by seeing a coronal section of the bone (Fig. 8.27). It consists of a midline *perpendicular plate*, two cuboidal bony masses on either side *(labyrinth)*, which are connected to the perpendicular plate by an horizontal *cribriform plate*.

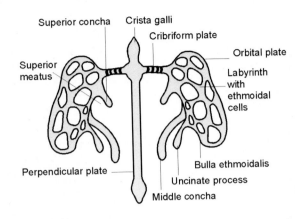

Fig. 8.27: Schematic diagram of coronal section through ethmoid

Perpendicular Plate

At the upper end of the perpendicular plate *crista galli* is present. The crista galli is seen in the floor of the anterior cranial cavity. The perpendicular plate takes part in the formation of the median nasal septum.

Labyrinths

The right and left labyrinths are fragile, pneumatic bone.
• It consists of many small air spaces *(ethmoidal air sinuses)*. The ethmoidal air sinuses are arranged in the anterior, middle and posterior groups.
• The walls of these air spaces are very thin and incomplete. The labyrinth is present between nasal and orbital cavities.
• The medial wall of the labyrinth is a part of the lateral wall of the nasal cavity and is bounded by the medial plate. From this medial plate there arises *superior and middle conchae*. Deep to middle concha there is

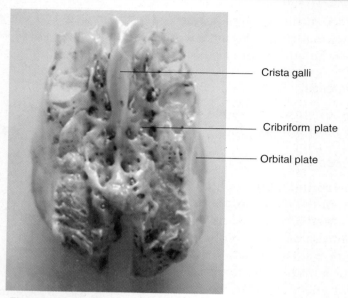

Fig. 8G: Superior aspect of ethmoid bone

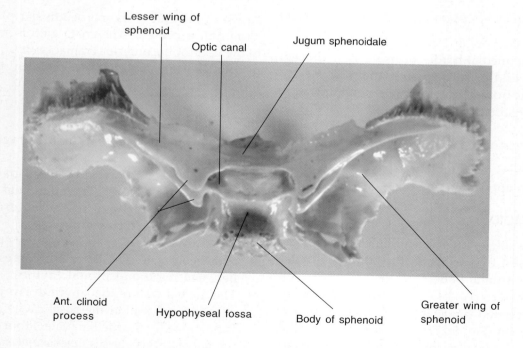

Fig. 8H: Superior aspect of sphenoid bone. Anterior clinoid process is bifid

the presence of a hook like *uncinate process* and a rounded elevation, the *bulla ethmoidale* (Fig. 7.43).

* The lateral wall of the labyrinth is formed by the orbital plate. The orbital plate forms the part of the medial wall of the orbit.

Cribriform Plate

The cribriform plate is the horizontal plate with numerous perforations. It connects the labyrinths with the median perpendicular plate. The cribriform plate is seen in the floor of the anterior cranial fossa on either side of crista galli. It also form the roof of the nasal cavity.

Articulations

* *Perpendicular plate* articulates with vomer, septal cartilage, frontal, nasal and sphenoid bone (Figs. 7.39 and 7.42).
* *Cribriform plate* articulates with the orbital plate and sphenoid bone.
* *Labyrinth* articulates with frontal, sphenoid, maxilla, lacrimal, perpendicular plate of palatine and inferior nasal concha (Fig. 7.43).

Ossification

The ethmoid bone ossifies in cartilagenous capsule. There appears three centres, i.e., one for perpendicular plate and one each for labyrinth. The centres for labyrinth appear in 4th month of IUL. The centre for perpendicular plate appears during first year of age. All centres unite to form a single bone by the end of third year of age.

PALATINE BONE

It is situated between maxilla and pterygoid process. It is L shaped in appearance and consists of perpendicular and horizontal plates. It also has three processes, i.e., pyramidal, orbital and sphenoidal (Fig. 8.28).

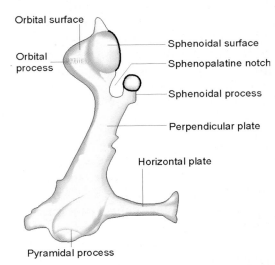

Fig. 8.28: Left palatine bone as seen from behind

Horizontal Plate

The horizontal plate forms the posterior part of hard plate. It shows a superior and an inferior surface. It has four borders, i.e., anterior, posterior, lateral and medial. The posterior border is free and projects backwards in the midline to form *posterior nasal spine.*

Perpendicular Plate

It has two surfaces, maxillary and nasal and four borders, i.e., anterior, posterior, superior and inferior. The maxillary or lateral surface shows the presence of a greater palatine groove, which is converted into greater palatine canal with the help of maxilla. This surface also forms the medial wall of the pterygopalatine fossa. The nasal (medial surface) has two horizontal crests (i.e., *ethmoidal crest*, which articulates with the middle concha of ethmoid bone and *conchal crest* articulates with the inferior concha).

The posterior border of the perpendicular plate articulates with the medial pterygoid plate. The superior border of perpendicular plate bears an orbital process and a sphenoidal process. Between these two process there is the presence of a *spheno-palatine notch,* which is converted into sphenopalatine foramen with the body of sphenoid.

Pyramidal Process

The pyramidal process is directed backwards and laterally from the junction of horizontal and perpendicular plates. This process fits into pterygoid fissure of pterygoid processes. Its inferior surface presents lesser palatine foramina.

Orbital Process

It is present at the anterior end of the upper border of perpendicular plate. It forms the posterior part of the floor of orbit.

Sphenoidal Process

It is situated at the posterior end of the upper border of the perpendicular plate. This process is grooved to complete the palatino-vaginal canal.

SPHENOID BONE

It is single, irregular, pneumatic bone situated posterior to the ethmoid and frontal bone. It forms the middle part of the base of the skull (Figs. 7.7, 7.24 and 7.34).

General Features

The sphenoid consists of:
- A centrally placed body.

- A pair of greater and lesser wings.
- The right and left pterygoid processes.

Body

The body of the sphenoid is cuboidal in shape and contains a pair of sphenoidal air sinus. It has six surfaces (i.e., *superior, inferior, anterior, posterior and right and left lateral surfaces*).

- The *superior surface* of the body bears the hypophyseal fossa. It forms the posterior part of the anterior cranial fossa (jugum sphenoidale, sulcus chiasmaticus and tuberculum sellae) and the central part of the middle cranial fossa (hypophyseal fossa, dorsum sellae and posterior clinoid process) (Fig. 7.34).
- The *inferior surface* of the body forms the posterior part of the roof of nasal cavity and the roof of nasopharynx. It shows a median ridge called as *rostrum*, which articulates with the grooved margin of vomer.
- The anterior surface of the sphenoid articulates with the ethmoid. It presents a median ridge called as *sphenoidal crest* for the articulation with the perpendicular plate of ethmoid bone. On either side of the crest lies a thin plate of bone called *sphenoidal concha*. The sphenoidal foramen lies above and medial to the concha.
- *Posterior surface* is rough and articulates with the basilar part of the occipital bone (Fig. 8.29).
- The upper part of the *lateral surface* is seen in the floor of the middle cranial fossa and shows a shallow groove the carotid sulcus. The lower part of the lateral surface unites with the greater wing and medial pterygoid plate.

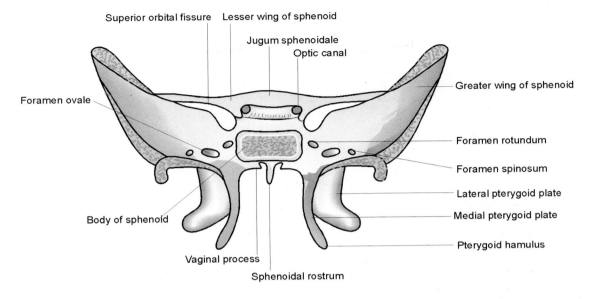

Superior orbital fissure   Lesser wing of sphenoid

Jugum sphenoidale
Optic canal

Greater wing of sphenoid

Foramen ovale

Foramen rotundum

Foramen spinosum

Lateral pterygoid plate

Medial pterygoid plate

Body of sphenoid

Pterygoid hamulus

Vaginal process

Sphenoidal rostrum

Fig. 8.29: The sphenoid bone

Wings

Greater Wings

Each greater wing has three surfaces, i.e., *cerebral (upper)*, *orbital* and *lateral*.

- The *cerebral surface* forms a part of the middle cranial fossa and related to the temporal lobe of cerebrum. Antero-medially, it has a sharp free margin, which forms the inferolateral boundary of the superior orbital fissure. This surface shows the presence of foramen rotundum, ovale and spinosum.

- The *lateral surface* of the greater wing of sphenoid is divided into upper temporal surface and lower infratemporal surface. The infratemporal surface forms the roof of infratemporal fossa. This surface shows the opening of foramen ovale and spinosum. This surface also shows the presence of the spine of sphenoid, which is present posterolateral to foramen spinosum. At the junction of temporal and infratemporal surface there is presence of *infratemporal crest*.

- The *orbital surface* is quadrilateral in shape and forms the part of the lateral wall of the orbit. This surface is in relation to the superior orbital fissure (above) and inferior orbital fissure (below).

Lesser Wings

It extends laterally from the anterosuperior part of the body of the sphenoid.

- It is connected to the body by anterior and posterior roots. In between two roots and body of sphenoid there is the presence of the *optic canal*.

- Lesser wing consists of two surfaces (*superior and inferior*) and two borders (*anterior and posterior*). The superior surface forms the posterior most part of the floor of the anterior cranial fossa. The inferior surface forms the superior border, of the superior orbital fissure.

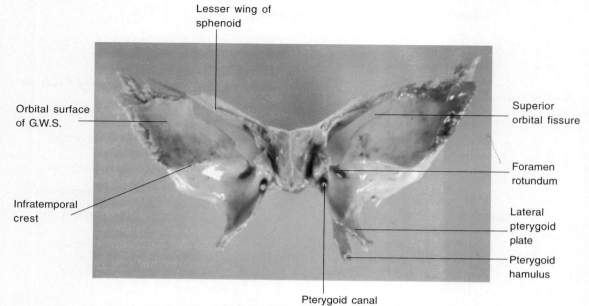

Lesser wing of sphenoid

Orbital surface of G.W.S.

Superior orbital fissure

Foramen rotundum

Infratemporal crest

Lateral pterygoid plate

Pterygoid hamulus

Pterygoid canal

Fig. 8I: Sphenoid bone as seen from anterior aspect

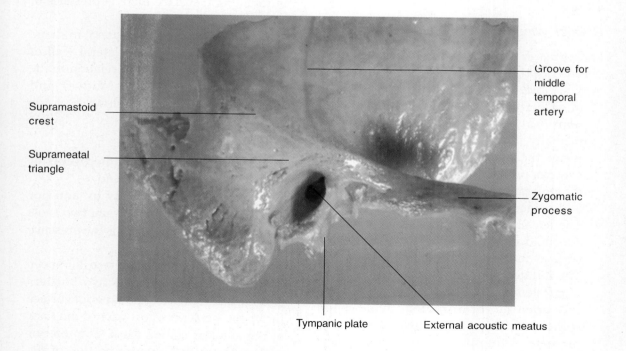

Groove for middle temporal artery

Supramastoid crest

Suprameatal triangle

Zygomatic process

Tympanic plate

External acoustic meatus

Fig. 8J: External surface of right temporal bone

- The anterior border articulates with the posterior border of the orbital plate, while posterior border is free.
- The medial end of the posterior border ends in the *anterior clinoid process.*

Pterygoid Processes

The pterygoid processes, on either side, extend downwards from the junction of the root of the greater wing and body of the sphenoid.
- Each process consists of lateral and medial pterygoid plates, which are separated posteriorly from each other by pterygoid fossa.
- Anteriorly both the plates are continuous with each other and form the posterior wall of pterygopalatine fossa.
- Following three foramina open anteriorly in the pterygoid process—foramen rotundum, pterygoid canal and palatino-vaginal canal.

Articulations

Body of sphenoid	Ethmoid bone (anteriorly), basilar part of the occipital (posteriorly)
Lesser wing of sphenoid	Orbital plate of frontal bone anteriorly
Greater wing of sphenoid	Frontal bone (antero-medially) Zygomatic bone (antero-laterally) Parietal bone (superiorly) Squamous temporal bone (posterolateral) Petrous temporal (posteriorly)
Pterygoid process	Maxilla (anteriorly) Perpendicular plate of palatine (Medial pterygoid plate).

Pyramidal process of palatine (Lower ends of pterygoid plates).

Ossification

The sphenoid gets ossified partly in membrane and partly in cartilage.

TEMPORAL BONE

The temporal bone is situated on each side of the base and side of the skull. This bone consists of the following parts:
- Squamous.
- Petrosal.
- Mastoid.
- Tympanic.
- Styloid process.

Squamous Part

It is thin plate like bone. It forms the antero-superior part of the bone. It has external (temporal) and internal (cerebral) surfaces and a superior and an anteroinferior border.
- The external surface (on the lateral aspect) shows the *zygomatic process, roots of the zygomatic process, supramastoid crest, temporal lines* and *supra-meatal triangle* (Figs. 8.30 and 8.31).
- The external surface (on the inferior aspect) is made up of a small *infratemporal surface, articular tubercle, mandibular fossa* and *squamotympanic fissure.*
- The internal or cerebral surface is concave and shows impression for the gyri of cerebrum and for blood vessels.

Mastoid Part

It lies posteroinferior to the squamous part. It shows external and internal surfaces and posterior border.

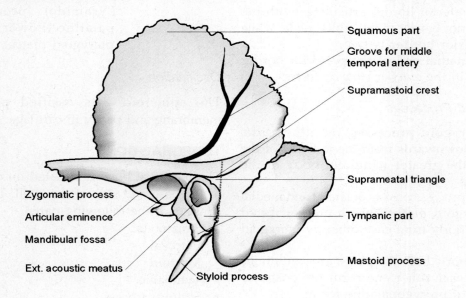

Squamous part

Groove for middle temporal artery

Supramastoid crest

Suprameatal triangle

Tympanic part

Mastoid process

Zygomatic process

Articular eminence

Mandibular fossa

Ext. acoustic meatus

Styloid process

Fig. 8.30: The lateral aspect of left temporal bone

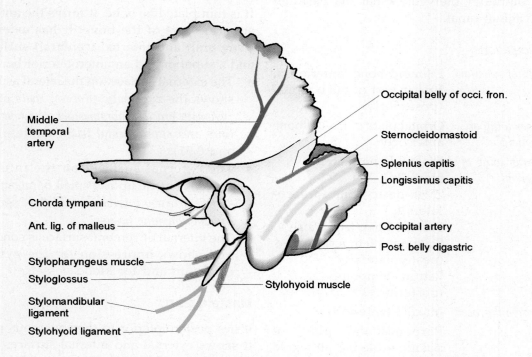

Occipital belly of occi. fron.

Sternocleidomastoid

Splenius capitis

Longissimus capitis

Middle temporal artery

Chorda tympani

Ant. lig. of malleus

Stylopharyngeus muscle

Styloglossus

Stylomandibular ligament

Stylohyoid ligament

Occipital artery

Post. belly digastric

Stylohyoid muscle

Fig. 8.31: Soft tissue relation of left temporal bone (external surface)

- It bears a downward extending conical projection, the mastoid process.
- The outer surface is smooth and may show the opening of mastoid foramen near its posterior border.
- The inner surface is marked by a vertical groove for the sigmoid sinus.
- The medial surface of the mastoid process shows a deep groove called the mastoid notch and a shallow groove for the occipital artery.

Petrous Part

This part of the bone is triangular in shape and present at the base of the skull. It has a base, an apex, three borders (superior, anterior and posterior) and three surfaces (anterior, posterior and inferior). The bone contains the internal and middle ear cavities.

Base

The base of the petrous bone is directed backwards and laterally and fuses with the squamous and mastoid parts.

Apex

It is directed forwards and medially. It forms the posterior margin of the foramen lacerum.

Borders

- The superior border demarcates the middle cranial fossa from the posterior cranial fossa. It is grooved by the superior petrosal sinus.
- The medial part of the anterior border articulates with the greater wing of the sphenoid and lateral part fuses with the squamous part.
- The medial part of the posterior border forms a sulcus for inferior petrosal sinus.

The lateral part forms the boundary of jugular foramen.

Surfaces

- The *anterior surface* of the petrous bone forms the posterior wall of the middle cranial fossa and shows the following features from medial to the lateral side—*trigeminal impression, hiatus for greater peetrosal nerve, hiatus for lesser petrosal nerve, arcuate imminence and tegmen tmympani.*
- The *posterior surface* forms the anterior wall of the posterior cranial fossa and shows the opening of internal acoustic meatus.
- The *inferior surface* of the petrous bone is rough and presents the lower opening of the carotid canal, depression of the jugular fossa in front of jugular foramen.

The Tympanic Part

It is curved plate of bone, situated anterior and inferior to the external acoustic meatus. It forms the non-articular posterior wall of the mandibular fossa.

This plate forms the anterior, inferior and lower part of the posterior wall of the external acoustic meatus.

The superior border of the tympanic plate meets the squamous temporal bone at the squamotympanic fissure. The inferior border forms a sheath for the base of styloid process. The rough lateral margin of the tympanic plate gives attachment to cartilaginous part the external acoustic meatus.

The Styloid Process

The styloid process is a conical projection of about 2.5 cm long. It is present on the inferior aspect of the temporal bone. It is directed downwards forwards and medially. The root of the styloid process is ensheathed by the tympanic plate. The stylomastoid foramen is situated between styloid and mastoid process.

Articulations

Squamous part - With greater wing of sphenoid anteriorly
With the parietal bone superiorly
With the head of mandible at tempo-romandibular joint

Petrous part - With the greater wing of sphenoid anteriorly

Mastoid part - With the occipital bone posteriorly
With the parietal bone superiorly
With the occipital bone posteriorly and medially

Zygomatic process - With the temporal process of zygomatic bone.

Side Determination and Anatomical Position

Hold the bone in such a way that:
- The zygomatic process faces anteriorly.
- External acoustic meatus laterally.
- The mastoid process faces backwards and downwards.

Ossification

Following parts of the bone ossify separately:

Part	Type of ossification	Appearance of center	Fusion
Squamous	Membranous (by single center)	2nd month of intrauterine life	All these centers
Tympanic	Membranous (by single center)	3rd month of intrauterine life	fuses with each
Petromastoid	Cartilaginous (by multiple centers)	5th month of intrauterine life	other by first year
Styloid	Cartilaginous (by two centers)	Just before birth	of life.

Further Readings

- Pal G.P. (1984). *Journal of Anatomy* (U.K.) 38 (2): 259-266.
- Pal G.P. (1987). *Journal of Anatomy* (U.K.) 152: 205-208.

INDEX